DIGESTIVE DISORDERS

[Common Issues]

DIGESTIVE DISORDERS

Common Issues

Dr. B.K. Agrawal

MBBS, MD (Medicine), DM (Gastroenterology), FICS

Dr. Pradip Kumar Agrawal

MBBS, MD (Medicine), MD (Radiology), FIAMS

RAJKAMAL PRAKASHAN

New Delhi Patna Allahabad

ISBN : 978-81-267-2085-9

Price: ₹ 125

First Edition: February, 2012
First Reprint: September, 2012

Published by:
Rajkamal Prakashan Pvt. Ltd.
1-B, Netaji Subhash Marg
New Delhi-110 002 (India)

Branches: Opposite Science College, Ashok Rajpath, Patna-800 006
First Floor, Darbari Building, M.G. Marg, Allahabad-211 001

Email: info@rajkamalprakashan.com
Website: www.rajkamalprakashan.com

Cover: Rajkamal Studio

Printed at:
B.K. Offset
Naveen Shahdara, Delhi-110 032

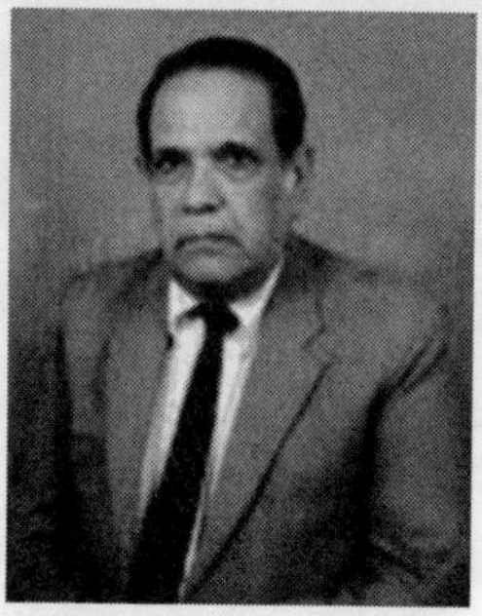

Professor (Dr.) B.N. Tandon
MBBS MD FAMS
Former Dean and Head of the department.
Gastroenterology, AIIMS, New Delhi
Former Chairman, Board of Directors, IGIMS, Patna.
Awarded Padma Bhushan by the President of India

GIFT OF KNOWLEDGE

This book on abdominal problems is written in quite simple language, so that everyone can understand easily. It is human nature to get attracted by the outside world and try to know about it. But we remain ignorant and careless about our own bodies. It is unfortunate that a common man does not even know the simple facts of human body. He does not try to understand the cause of a medical problem and thinks that, 'A pill is good for every ill'.

The symptoms of frequently encountered abdominal problems are discussed by Dr. B. K. Agrawal and Dr. P. K. Agrawal in a lucid manner. The knowledge may immensely benefit a common man. Knowledge displaces ignorance, as the light replaces darkness. The public should have the knowledge about health and diseases for their own personal well being. Good health is the greatest wealth for an individual, which can be attained by knowing about our body systems, diseases and various options of treatment. A healthy person should know how to stay fit and healthy. An ill person should try to understand his disease and should explore various methods to obtain cure.

In our country the awareness of the general public regarding health is quite dismal. Such books may help in improving the level of knowledge and awareness.

In my opinion charity of money is good, charity of food is better, however the charity of knowledge is the best and the greatest.

The initiative to educate people and the charity of knowledge by the authors is highly commendable.

Prof. (Dr.) B.N. Tandon

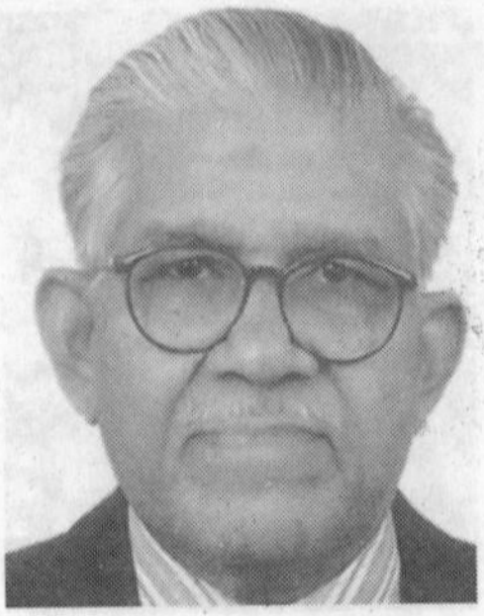

Dr. (Prof.) Shyam Narayan Arya
MBBS (Hons. & Gold Medalist), MD (Pat.)
FRCP (Edin.), FRCP (Glassg.), FCCP (USA)
FICA (USA), FNCCP (Ind.).), FIAMS (Ind.). FICP (Ind.)
FIACM (Ins.)
Ex-National Professor of Medicine and Dean of Studies, IMA College of G.P.
Dr. B.C. Roy National Awardee
Awarded Padmshree by the President of India

BOOK WITH A MESSAGE

I have read this book written by Dr. Brij Kishore Agrawal and Dr. Pradip Kumar Agrawal from the beginning to the end. Dr. B.K. Agrawal is a renowned gastroenterologist of national fame. Dr. P.K. Agrawal is a well known physician and radiologist.

People nurture many myths, misconceptions and doubts about abdominal diseases. The book clears all such doubts. It answers frequently asked questions in easy and simple language. Detailed discussions of various symptoms of abdominal diseases, ways to avoid them and diet in abdominal diseases are the highlights of the book.

A very important message is given in this book, that to call a doctor at home for consultation is nothing more than a 'status symbol' in modern medical practices. This principle applies equally well to diseases of any and every body system. A doctor at home visit cannot achieve much if the patient is having a heart attack. A sick patient should always be transferred to a hospital for proper care.

The objective of the book is to tell practical things to a common man. It is not aimed at making him a quack. The book does not prescribe medicines, but gives life-style tips to avoid abdominal problems. The book stands well with its stated objectives.

Several books have been written by non-medical professionals on health topics. However, there was a noticeable dearth of reliable books based on scientific facts and written by doctors. This book fulfils the gap nicely.

Authors of the book deserve all the accolades on writing such a reader friendly book on a medical topic.

Dr. S.N. Arya

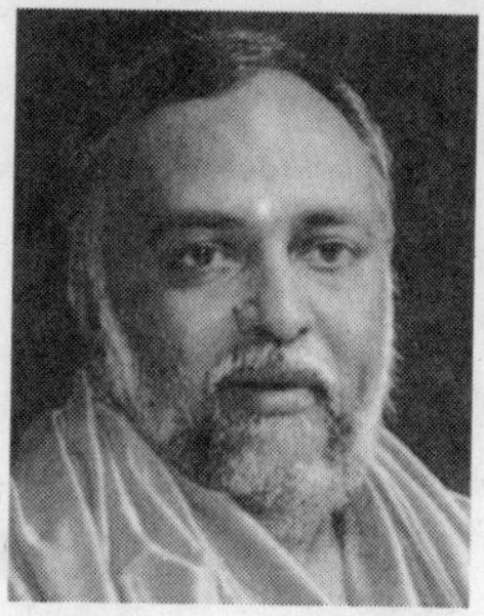

Swami Sukhabodhananda
Founder Chairman
Prasanna Trust, Banglore
www.swamisukhabodhananda.org
email: prasannatrust@vsnl.com

I wish and pray that authors' valuable insights in medical science will help humanity for a better healthy living.

At a time where high technological medicines have had innumerable side effects, it becomes really essential for people like you, to explore into alternative, healing methods. This search for better healing methods and using local wisdom is a part of wise living. One should never give up this endeavour.

One should always be aware that mind can play an influential role in self-healing. It is said that 75% of snakebites are non poisonous and most of the time people fear or even die when a non-poisonous snake bites a person. So it is clear that mind plays a strong role in shaping an individual.

There has also been an onset of what is called "energy medicines". When a person is angry, jealous…certain negative energies are released which is not good for one's health. But when a person operates through love, kindness, positivity…a different form of energy is released in an individual and such energies helps in healing process.

All these alternative medicines are now a formidable force in health care because it has its roots traditionally from the grass root levels with a single objective of love to heal. I pray that this book will help you to demystify the complexities and simplify the way to use alternative and healthy ways to heal oneself.

Always understand that every alternate medicine has healing properties and when rightly used with a deep commitment then the best results would happen. I wish that this book will create a wise way to heal oneself. I appreciate the effort put by you and wish you all the best in reaching many.

With Blessings
Swami Sukhabodhananda

ACKNOWLEDGMENT

Our first book on abdominal problem in Hindi, 'PET-ROG' (Vyaavharik Baatein) was well appreciated by everyone and it was tremendously successful commercially. Many readers felt a need and recommended a similar 'easy-to-learn' book with simple language in English. Our first and foremost thank goes to Shri Ashok Maheshwari, who appreciated the need, encouraged us to write and published it in a short span of time.

We express our sincere gratitude to Shree Vivekanand Ojha, a teacher of Biology in Sudarshan Central School, Patna and Shree Om Prakash Choudhry a teacher of English in the same school for secreening and correcting the manuscript

We thank Dr. Anant Kumar Singh and Dr. Sanjeev Kumar, consultants at Agrawal Gastroentrology and Liver clinic, Patna for their useful suggestions, We are thankful to Shree Gautam Prakash for internet services. We thank Shri Dharmender Vishwakarma for typing the manuscript and preparing the initial layout.

Smt. Anjali Agrawal, W/O Dr. B.K. Agrawal and Smt. Meenu Agrawal, W/O Dr. P.K. Agrawal deserve special mention for their encouragement and support.

Ravi, Shalini and Shivani, children of Dr. B.K. Agrawal; and Prashant and Rishab, children of Dr. P.K. Agrawal have contributed to these projects by making our lives happy and purposeful.

Authors

CONTENT

CHAPTER-1

• PAIN ABDOMEN

The marriage of engineer son of Mr. Kumar was celebrated last evening. It was a gala event with music, dance and dinner. He along with his entourage came back to his house late in the night. Early in the morning he is having severe pain in his belly. Medical help is out of reach at present. The question hovering in his mind is, whether is it a simple discomfort out of overeating and exertion or is it some serious matter like appendicitis or heart attack?

Pain in abdomen, the main symptom of abdominal diseases is caused by a variety of problems. On one hand it may be due to simple things, like overeating, worms or mental tension and on the other hand it may signify something serious, such as stone in the gall bladder or in the kidneys. We know that correct diagnosis only can lead to correct treatment of medical problems. To make a correct assessment of seriousness of abdominal pain is quite challenging task for the attendants as well as the doctors.

SIGNS OF SERIOUSNESS

To find whether the pain is a serious matter and warrants prompt attention, the following points should be looked into :

1. **Severity of the pain -** Whether the abdominal pain is intense making him uncomfortable with grimacing and restlessness. Severe pain suggests some serious problem.

2. **Nausea & Vomiting -** Whether he is having nausea, the unpleasant feeling as if he is about to vomit? Whether he is vomiting?
3. **Guarding of Abdomen -** The abdomen feels hard on touch due to contraction of muscles in abdominal wall.
4. **Fever -** Is he febrile, having mouth temperature above 100°F?
5. **Giddiness -** Is he experiencing weakness, exhaustion and giddiness? Is he sweating?

The association of any one of the above mentioned symptoms along with severe abdominal pain suggests a potentially life threatening condition. This set of symptoms is called 'Acute Abdomen' in medical language. The condition of the patient in such condition may worsen rapidly. 'Acute Abdomen' requires prompt work up, as accurate diagnosis is needed for proper treatment. Whether he requires any surgical intervention or not, also needs to be answered. The sufferer may need hospitalisation for proper medical care.

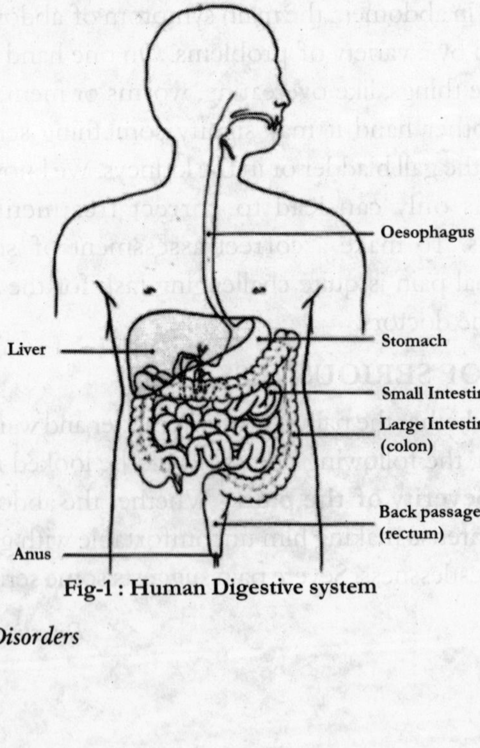

Fig-1 : Human Digestive system

The location of the pain and its spread help doctors in finding its cause and the affected organ. Upper abdominal pain is generally related to the organs of the digestive system like liver, kidneys, stomach, gall bladder and pancreas. Pain around umbilicus suggests disease in small intestines and appendix. Pain in the lower abdomen may be due diseases of colon, urinary bladder and the other organs in pelvis.

Severe abdominal pain may be harbinger of abdominal diseases as well as that of the lungs (Pleurisy) and the heart (Heart Attack). The actual cause can only be found by clinical work up and investigations.

The practice of modern medicine requires teamwork by doctors, nurses and laboratory technicians. It also necessitates the use of imaging equipments to take pictures of abdominal organs for analysis. Ultrasonography has emerged as the first and most important imaging modality in the work up of pain abdomen. Home visit by a doctor is generally not very helpful in such a situation. We must realize that it is better to take the patient with pain abdomen to a well equipped clinic or hospital.

When the abdominal pain is not associated with the "signs of seriousness", some home remedies like antispasmodic or antacid may be tried. If pain is not relieved in 1-3 hours, the doctor should be consulted.

The fact that practitioners of modern medicine are generally not able to help much at home visit cannot be overemphasized. Whether it is abdominal pain, vomiting, breathlessness or chest pain, all require medical services in a clinic and hospital setup, where diagnostic and support systems are available.

If the condition is serious it is unwise to call the doctor at home. On the other hand, if the problem is not serious, the home visit by doctor is a nothing more than a 'status symbol'. If you have a family physician you may contact him to help you reach the right doctor at the right place, as clinics and hospitals also are specialized giving services to specific medical problems.

CAUSES OF ABDOMINAL PAIN

Two body systems are located inside the abdominal cavity:

1. **Digestive System** - It includes organ like stomach, duodenum, intestines, liver, gall bladder and pancreas which are involved in digesting, assimilating and storing food.
2. **Genito-urinary system** - Kidneys, Ureters and urinary bladder are the organs which excrete byproducts of metabolism in the urine

In women, additionally the Reproductive system, comprising of uterus, ovaries and fallopian tubes, is located in the abdomen.

It is quite natural that majority of the patients of pain abdomen would have afflictions of the systems mentioned.

Certain important and frequent causes of abdominal pain are briefly described:-

(1) Gall Bladder Stone - Liver produces bile, a digestive juice, which is stored in a sac known as gall bladder. The stored bile is released in duodenum on arrival of food, where it helps in digestion of fat.

During storage of the bile sometimes the crystals precipitate out of liquid and form sand like particles, which by clumping and further deposition of crystals on it, become stones.

In our country about one in every two hundred persons may probably have gall bladder stone during his lifetime. At a given time only 10% of persons having gall stone in a population have noticeable symptoms.

The presence of stones in the gall bladder generally cause gas, distension of abdomen and discomfort on taking fatty food. The movement of the stone in the gall bladder causes pain, known as biliary colic, which is generally quite severe and may spread to entire abdomen or towards the right shoulder.

When the stone gets impacted at the narrow neck portion of the gall bladder (figure-2) the outflow of the bile is blocked, gall bladder distends and acute abdominal pain ensues. The condition in medical terminology is called 'Acute Cholecystitis', in which severe pain in right upper part of the abdomen is accompanied by vomiting and fever. This pain can be felt in chest, right shoulder or back as well.

The treatment of the gall stone disease is surgery, in which entire gall bladder along with stones is taken out. Surgery is advised for the following reasons:

A. The stone may cause recurrent pain due to swelling of the gall bladder (Cholecystitis).

B. If the stone passes to bile duct it may cause jaundice, colic, itching and at times inflammation of the pancreas (Pancreatitis).

C. Gall Bladder stone is thought to be associated with cancer of the gall bladder which has high incidence in the transgangetic belt of India.

Majority of the gall bladder stones in western population are cholesterol stones in nature which may remain silent throughout life of the person. Compared to this in Indian population, most of the gall bladder stones are mixed stones in composition indicating infective cause, which may be the reason for high incidence of cancer like changes.

Surgical excision of gall bladder today has become easy and convenient with the advent of Laparoscopic technique, also known as 'key-hole' surgery. In the past gall bladder used to be

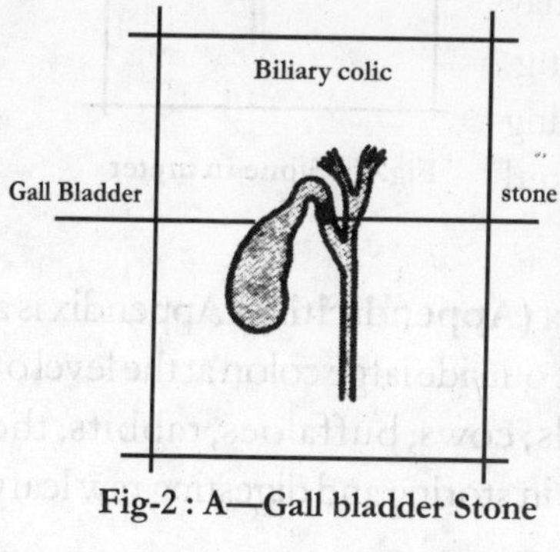

Fig-2 : A—Gall bladder Stone

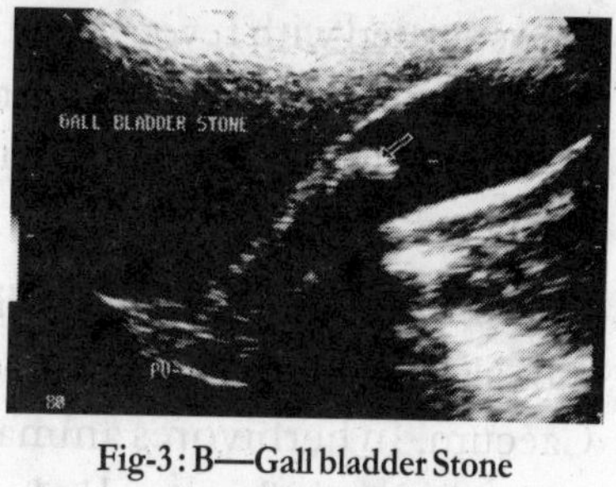

Fig-3 : B—Gall bladder Stone (Ultrasound Image)

operated by making a 5-10cms cut over the wall of the abdomen. In the key-hole surgery, only 3-4 small holes (ports) are made through which pipe like light source and long handle instruments are introduced to remove the diseased organ.

This type of surgery is also called 'minimal invasive surgery' as there is very small amount of blood loss and tissue injury. The period of stay at the hospital is also short in key-hole surgery. The new laparoscopy technique involves using expensive equipment thereby increasing the cost of the surgery, however overall cost including the bill for the hospital stay and medicines is almost similar.

(2) Stones in the Urinary Tract (Kidneys, Ureters & Urinary Bladder) - Kidney, the key organ of excretory system filters out the harmful byproducts of metabolism, urea and creatinine from the blood and excretes these waste matters in the urine. Various other waste chemicals like oxalate, calcium, phosphate and uric acid also generally remain dissolved in urine. If the urine gets concentrated, these chemicals precipitate forming crystals that lead to stone formation.

Movement of a stone from kidney through ureter to urinary bladder causes severe pain termed 'uretric colic' which classically spreads from 'loin to groin'. The pain of stone of urinary system may be associated with fever, vomiting, reddish urine (Haematuria), burning in urine (Dysuria) and increased frequency of urine.

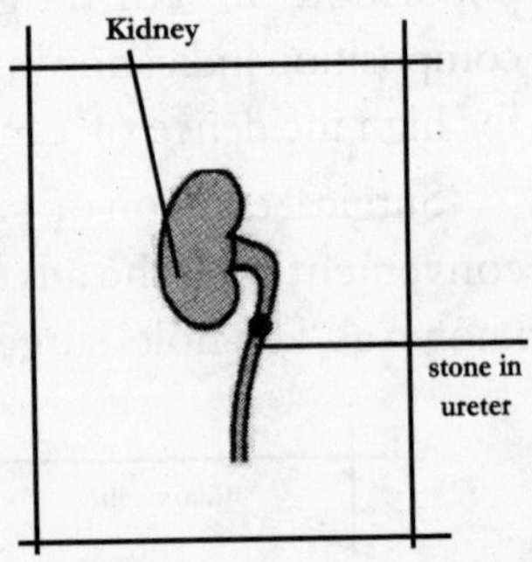

Fig.-4 : Stone in ureter

(3) Inflammation of Appendix (Appendicitis) - Appendix is a tube like blind pouch of intestine outside large colon at the level of Caecum. In herbivores animals; cows, buffaloes, rabbits, the appendix is quite large and helps in storing and digesting raw leafy food. It is quite small in human beings and is considered to have lost its utility (Vestigial organ).

As appendix is a blind tube any blockage of its opening due to seed, food or worm, causes its dilatation and swelling. The bacteria grow in the dilated appendix, resulting in its inflammation—**Acute Appendicitis.** The pain of appendicitis begins around navel and moves towards right lower part of the abdomen. It is usually associated with vomiting and fever.

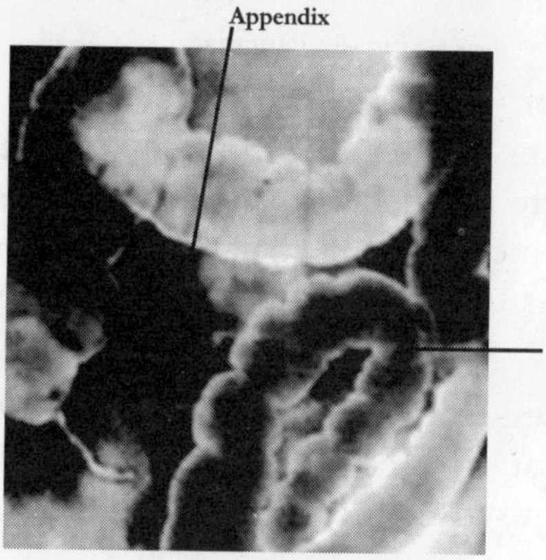

Fig.-5 : Appendix and colon

Appendicitis initially is generally treated with antibiotics followed by surgery. Occasionally emergency surgery may be required if the inflammation is severe and if there is possibility of perforation of appendix.

(4) Inflammation of Pancreas (Pancreatitis) - Pancreas, an organ situated behind stomach, produces insulin the hormone which controls blood sugar level. It also produces pancreatic enzymes which helps in the digestion of fat.

Main causes of the inflammation of pancreas are ingestion of alcohol and presence of stones in the gall bladder. Injury to abdomen by a blow of fist, handle of bicycle, steering wheel also may cause Pancreatitis.

Acute Pancreatitis causes pain in upper abdomen that spreads to back. It is a serious and life threatening condition, warranting immediate medical attention.

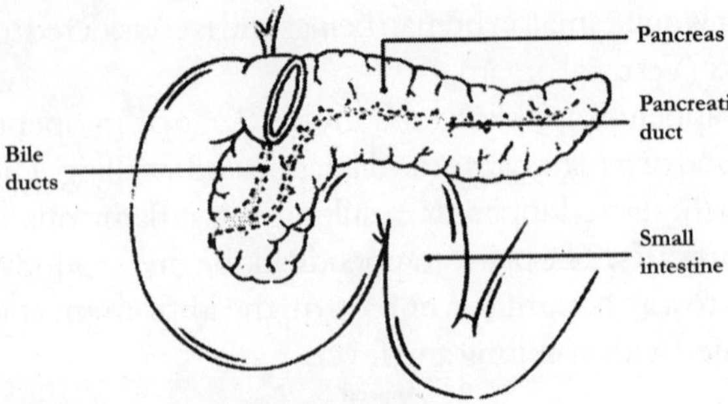

Fig.-6 : Pancreas

(5) Peptic Ulcer - Increased amount of acid in stomach and duodenum causes ulcers in the inner lining of these organs, known as peptic ulcer. Peptic ulcer causes pain in upper abdomen. The ulcer may bleed causing vomiting of coffee ground vomitus or making the stool black and tar-like in appearance.

(6) Pain Related to Female Reproductive Organs - The inflammation of ovaries (Oophritis) and fallopian tubes (Salpingitis), caused by infection are painful conditions in women.

Many young women suffer pain in lower abdomen in the beginning of menstruation or during the period of bleeding. The release of egg from the ovary (Ovulation) may also cause pain. The pain of ovulation occurs in the period between two menstrual cycles (Mid-cycle pain).

The pains related to reproductive organs are analysed and treated by a gynecologist.

Sometimes the pain related to heart (Heart-attack) and chest (Pneumonia, Pleurisy) may spread to upper part of the abdomen confusing the doctors. The pain of heart problem generally increases with effort and gets relieved on resting. At times persons with 'Angina' may present with 'gas' or upper abdominal discomfort.

It is reiterated that abdominal pain requires thorough clinical work-up and investigations to arrive at correct diagnosis and guiding proper management.

CHAPTER-2

• NAUSEA AND VOMITING

Vomiting is the process of forceful expulsion of the contents of the stomach through mouth. Vomiting is generally preceded by nausea, which is an unpleasant subjective feeling of impending vomiting. A nauseated person only initiates the act of vomiting but does not complete it.

Causes

A variety of things, smells, food stuffs etc may make someone nauseous. Unpleasant food, rotting garbage, carcass, hospital smells, seeing blood and a variety of stimuli may cause nausea. Apart from the external stimuli, unpleasant food in the stomach and certain medical problems such as fever, migraine, epilepsy and diseases of the brain may also cause nausea and vomiting.

Overeating, spicy food and alcohol consumption may cause nausea and vomiting. Certain medicines like painkillers, especially when taken on empty stomach may cause edema and inflammation of internal lining (mucosa) of stomach (gastritis) leading to nausea, vomiting and bleeding from stomach wall.

Pregnant women, especially during first three months (first trimester) of pregnancy may suffer nausea and vomiting due to changes in hormones in the body. Occasionally the vomiting during pregnancy may be very severe and prolonged enough to make a woman miserable.

Nausea and vomiting may accompany some serious disease. Sometimes, an obstruction in the passage of food beyond stomach or small intestine may cause vomiting. The obstruction may be caused by spasm of the intestinal muscle, round worms in lumen of the gut or tumor in its wall.

Vomiting may be an associated symptom in many conditions causing abdominal pain, such as gall bladder stone, kidney stone, appendicitis and Pancreatitis etc. If a patient of vomiting is also having pain in the chest, perspiration, weakness and feeling of heaviness over heart, it may suggest heart attack, requiring immediate medical care in a hospital setup.

Vomiting along with headache, particularly in morning hours may be a pointer of high blood pressure or an attack of migraine. Sometimes an attack of paralysis (Stroke) in an elderly person is preceded by vomiting. An elderly person having slightest evidence of weakness in the limbs should get immediate medical attention, so that progression of the disease may be checked or minimized.

Effect of Vomiting

Vomiting causes loss of fluid and salt from the body, which leads to weakness and exhaustion. If the vomiting is profuse and prolonged the person may become dehydrated. Passing of small amounts of high colored urine, giddiness and extreme weakness are signs of dehydration, which is a medical emergency requiring immediate medical attention.

Blood in Vomitus

The presence of red colored fresh blood or brown, coffee-ground old blood in vomitus is a warning signal of some serious problem. Fresh blood in stomach becomes brownish after a few hours due to chemical reactions with gastric acids.

Ulcers in the stomach known as peptic ulcers are one of the most common causes of blood in vomitus. Excessive use of pain killers (Non-Steroidal-Anti-Inflammatory drugs like aspirin, Ibuprofen, nimuselide etc) may cause mucosal edema (Gastritis) and ulcers in stomach.

Bleeding from the nose or blood-mixed sputum may sometimes be ingested and later on expelled out as blood mixed vomitus. This sequence of events should be clearly understood, as here the disease is in the nose or lungs and not in the stomach. Therefore, the diagnostic approach and treatment should proceed accordingly.

While vomiting one should not try to check it forcibly. The act of vomiting involves contraction of abdominal and diaphragmatic muscles. An attempt to stop vomiting may stretch the junction of stomach with food pipe (Gastro-esophageal junction), tearing it, causing bleeding and its appearance in vomitus.

Some persons try to induce vomiting by putting fingers in the throat. This practice should be avoided as the acidic fluid of stomach may damage inner lining of food pipe and throat. The acid also reacts with calcium of teeth and may in long term damage them. Repeated acid reflux may lead to change in voice also.

FIRST AID in Nausea and Vomiting

The aims of first aid is first to control it and then replenish the fluid and salt lost in vomiting.

The nauseous feeling triggered by some flavors, smell or sight can naturally be relieved by getting away from that stimulus. Sucking ice-cube, sipping fluid (water, lemon etc) of someone's choice and taking antacid with water in a person having associated hyperacidity may reduce nausea. However when nausea is preceding vomiting, it may be worth while to let the content of stomach be expelled out, which most of the times settles the matter. Here the vomiting achieves the goal of the stomach to get rid of harmful substances.

The fluid lost in vomiting should be replaced by ingesting plain water, glucose solution, lemon water and oral rehydration solution etc. The fluid should be taken in small sips rather than in large gulps which may again provoke vomiting. In the beginning milk, soups and fizzy drinks should be avoided. If one feels better with the taste of a particular fizzy drink, it may be sipped after the fizz has bubbled out.

One may begin solid foods when the bouts of vomiting are controlled and fluids are retained by the body. Easily digestible carbohydrates, Rice, *Khichri, Moong-dal* and fresh curd are accepted by the body. Gradually protein in the form of milk and other pulses are added, leaving the fat containing food (*Puree, Paratha,* Sweets and spicy vegetables) for last on recovery.

CHAPTER-3

• CONSTIPATION

Constipation indicates inability to empty bowel easily and without straining. In other words passage of hard stool at less than desired frequency is expressed by people as constipation. The inability to get rid of faeces, which actually is residual unabsorbed food, leads to distension of the abdomen and a distressing sensation of bloating.

One should know the process of digestion in order to understand constipation. The ingested food is first broken to smaller pieces by chewing in the mouth and then ground to minute particle form by the peristaltic movements of the stomach. It is mixed with a variety of digestive juices such as saliva in mouth, gastric juice in stomach and bile and pancreatic juices in duodenum. The activity of the enzymes present in these juices breaks down the large molecules of protein, fat and carbohydrate into small and simple molecules of amino acids, saccharides and fatty acids etc, which get absorbed in small intestine. The residual unabsorbed food which mainly consists of dietary fibers is passed to colon where water is absorbed making the faeces solid in consistency. The faeces thus formed is stored in colon and shed outside through anus at regular intervals.

Statistical scientific studies have shown great variation in the frequency of bowel movements in population. It has been found to vary from three times a day to three times a week in normal people. The frequency of bowel movement depends upon individual characteristics like physical activity, mental status, the motility of the intestines and on the diet which someone is consuming.

In our part of world, people take greater quantity of dietary fibers, have bulkier stool and higher frequency of bowel movement. In western countries where people consume small quantity of very refined foods like biscuits, breads, jams, juices etc, pass smaller quantity of stool with lesser frequency. Constipation, a common problem afflicting about ten percent people in our population may thus be said to be present,

1. When the frequency of bowel emptying is less than three times a week.
2. When the person takes more than ten minutes to empty bowel.
3. When the stool is hard and dry.
4. When one has to strain and make extra effort to pass stool.

We must appreciate that apart from really constipated people, a large number of people have false notion of bowel movement and unduly worry about their bowel habits. The inability to pass clear stools twice a day is considered a sign of ill health in rural India. Many people go to toilet five-six times a day and still claim to be constipated.

Who Gets Constipated?

Physical activity in the form of walking and exercises is essential for good bowel movement. Persons having sedentary jobs, like office workers, businessmen and clerks find difficulty in emptying bowel easily.

Elderly people with waning muscular strength also have weak activity of intestinal muscles, making them constipated. The digestion of food is an active process demanding work by the digestive tract.

Sometimes in aged and bedridden persons the stool accumulates and dries up in the large colon. It irritates the inner lining of gut causing watery discharge and passage of watery stool. This misleading condition is termed 'Spurious diarrhoea'. Here one has to treat the constipation and take out the hard stool (Faecolith) accumulated near anus, manually or by giving enema. The treatment of spurious diarrhoea by anti diarrheal drugs may further worsen the condition.

Pregnant women also find it difficult to empty bowel, due to hormonal changes in the body and pressure of the gravid uterus over the rectum. Patients who have undergone surgery over abdomen and around anus may suffer from constipation.

A good bowel habit generally develops on its own during childhood. Children who are asked to sit at toilet pot regularly in the morning develop a reflex which empties the bowel at the fixed time. The activities of the body have an inner rhythm or a clock. Those children, whose body gets tuned for bowel emptying, generally maintain the habit in adult life. We should aim at going to toilet at a fixed time in the morning. The toilet training in the childhood has a lifetime impact on bowel movement.

Effects of Constipation

Constipation generally leads to gas formation, abdominal bloating and lack of interest in food. The person becomes irritable and lethargic. He may suffer from abdominal pain and headache. Sometimes the headache may be so uncomfortable that patient may claim, 'The gas has gone to head'.

Causes of Constipation

The life style factors that lead to constipation in otherwise healthy persons are:

A. Lack of Physical Activity.

B. Lack of fibre in diet.

C. Inadequate ingestion of water and other liquids.

Constipation is a prominent feature in a many medical conditions. Certain diseases of abdomen such as, Intestinal tuberculosis, 'Irritable Bowel Syndrome' (P-97), diseases of colon (Diverticulum) and anorectal area (Fissures, fistula, Hemorrhoids) may also cause constipation.

Constipation may be a dominant feature in a few endocrine diseases and the patient may clinically present with this symptom. Constipation may be a prominent symptom in Hypothyroidism- the deficiency of the thyroid hormone. Diseases of nervous system i.e. Parkinson's disease, and paralysis may lead to constipation. Certain medicines, like cough syrup (containing codeine), Antacids (Aluminium Hydroxide), pain killers of opium group and drugs given for psychiatric illness may also cause constipation.

Danger signs in constipation:

Constipation in itself is not very harmful, however when it is associated with fever, loss of weight, vomiting and blood in stool, it raises the possibility of some ongoing abdominal disease process. Such patients should consult a physician and undergo thorough medical checkup to find out the cause of constipation and associated symptoms.

Laxative, the medicines given for constipation act on intestine in many ways:-

A. Prokinetic agents (Mosapride, Itopride, domperidone, cinitapride etc) increase the motility of gut.

B. Contact laxatives (Bisacodyl, senna) irritate the colonic mucosa and stimulate them to move.

C. Bulk laxatives like Ispaghula husk contain fiber and increase the bulk of the stool.

D. Liquid paraffin softens the faeces.

E. Osmotic Laxative (Lactulose and lactitol) draws water from gut lining and softens the stool.

When the constipation is quite severe (Obstipation) the patient may need enema. In enema, plain water or medicated fluid is introduced through rectum to stimulate and clean the gut.

Long term use of Laxatives should be avoided as the person becomes dependent on them. Gradually the medicines lose their effect and larger doses may be needed to have the desired effect. Laxatives should be taken only on prescription by a doctor

Green leafy vegetables, fruits, full bran wheat, puffed rice, red gram and maize-flour are rich in fibre. These fibres help in giving bulk and softness to the stool, thereby allowing easy bowel clearance. They stimulate the intestine to move faster .High fibre food; adequate water intake and physical activity promote good bowel clearance and relieve constipation.

Box-1

Ways to Avoid Constipation

Do's:-

- Do physical exercises regularly. Walking, Jogging, Yoga, aerobics all are helpful. Use stairs and avoid lifts. Get involved in household chores like cleaning, washing cloths etc.
- Drink adequate water and liquids like fruit juices and soup etc.
- Take your food - Breakfast, Lunch, evening tea and dinner at scheduled time as far as practical
- Eat sumptuous breakfast- you need energy for the first shift of work.
- Eat relaxingly chewing every bolus at least 15 times
- Take plenty of fruits and vegetables in food.
- Go to toilet for bowel clearance at fixed time everyday. Your body clock will set accordingly.

Do Not's

- Do not ignore the urge to pass stool. The call of nature should be attended urgently.
- Do not be in a hurry in toilet.
- Avoid fried and fatty foods.
- Avoid strong tea, toast, banana and boiled egg when you are constipated.
- Do not take medications without doctor's advice.
- Avoid unnecessary fasting and practice of irregular eating.

CHAPTER- 4

• DIARRHOEA

Diarrhoea is the passage of frequent, loose and watery stools. When stool is mixed with blood the condition is called dysentery. Diarrhoea associated with vomiting is termed as gastroenteritis.

Diarrhoea, dysentery and Gastroenteritis are most of the times caused by the infection of the gut by micro-organisms. A variety of organisms, viruses, bacteria and protozoa enter our body along with contaminated food and water and invade the mucosa, i.e. the inner lining of gut. The infection leads to swelling of the inner lining which begins shedding large quantities of fluid, thereby causing passage of watery stools.

Certain medicines like Ampicilin and magnesium hydroxide antacids may also cause diarrhea. Diarrhoea in the true sense is attempt by the body to get rid of harmful microbes. The intestinal mucosa by increasing its secretions tries to wash it off. Generally the bouts of loose motions stop on its own within a few days. In majority of the patients it does not matter much whether medicines to check diarrhea is given a not. The only important and critical fact is that with fluid stools, large quantity of water and salts are lost from the body, which leads to dehydration and exhaustion. The loss of water and salt should be replaced quickly. Occasionally due to factors like duty, work or social events, it becomes essential to check diarrhoea, when medicines for symptomatic relief may be given.

WAYS TO AVOID DIARRHOEA

WATER

The first and foremost thing is to use clean and uncontaminated water for drinking purpose and preparing food.

The most important point is to take care of the source of the water. If the source is very dirty and the water coming out is heavily contaminated, all the efforts to purify it will have limited success. The water drawn from deep tube wells is generally free from harmful organisms. The water thus drawn should be stored in clean tanks and vessels. We remember to clean the drums and buckets in our houses but forget to regularly clean the overhead tanks, where water is stored for quite long time.

The large size water storage tanks in schools, buildings, offices and hospitals etc should be constructed with good quality material and cleaned every month, followed by chlorination of the water. The tank should always be kept covered to keep dust away.

The plastic tanks of many brands should be dark in colour. White and transparent tanks allow entry of light and promote the growth of algae in water.

The water should be made cleaner by letting it pass through Water filter, Aquaguard or a RO system (Reverse Osmosis System). Boiling the water may kill majority of the microbes, however it alters the taste of water. Boiling water for the requirement of all the members of a household in India, where majority are big joint families, may prove quite cumbersome and is impractical.

The purified water should be stored in clean vessels and bottles. Generally it remains potable for 2-3 hours at room temperatures and 4-6 hours if kept in the refrigerator.

FOOD

The main sources of infection in food items are fruits, salads and chutneys. Fruits and salads are good for health however, unlike rice, bread etc, these are eaten raw and uncooked. Varieties of bacteria reside on the surface of fruits and salads, which should be removed by thorough cleaning and rinsing in clean water.

Varieties of insecticides are sprayed on fruits and vegetable when these are in field and in store house. Thorough washing is essential to remove these residual amounts of insecticides before consuming fruits etc.

The prepared food should never be left uncovered, as flies and cockroaches can contaminate them. Eating from road side stalls selling fruits and chats should be avoided as far as possible.

Bottled and canned juice should be taken after pouring them in clean glass. The caps of bottles and juices generally become dirty and occasionally rusty during storage.

A housewife or the cook should prepare the food in quantity adequate for a particular breakfast, lunch or dinner depending upon the food habits of family member. In this way there will not be need to store leftover food and necessity to consume stale food.

The bacteria grow even in food kept in fridge, albeit a bit slowly. Boiled potato, milk, paneer etc are more liable to become infected even when kept at low temperatures. The food kept in fridge should always be warmed again before eating to kill harmful bacteria grown during storage.

UTENSILS

Utmost care should be taken to keep the kitchen and utensils clean. The cloth used to dry the utensils should also be clean. It should be washed regularly and changed frequently.

The peelings and seeds of fruits and vegetables and the food left in the plate should be put in a covered dust bin. Bacteria, virus and protozoa grow profusely over vegetative items and get transferred by flies, mosquitoes and cockroaches to our food.

The hands should be washed thoroughly before cooking food. If there is any cut or boil on hands or fingers it should be properly bandaged and wet work should be avoided.

Decorative crokeries if used at special occasions should be washed with plain water before putting them on the dining table to remove the dirt accumulated during storage.

Home Management of Diarrhoea

The fluid lost in watery stool should first be replenished by drinking plain water, lemon-water or coconut water. Packets of ORS powder dissolved in boiled and cooled water should be administered.

'Dahi ka Matha'

The thin watery preparation of curd replenishes lost water and salt in diarrhoea. It also introduces useful organism lactobacilli in gut, which replaces harmful Coliform bacteria.

A person suffering from diarrhoea should initially get easily digestible food. *Khichri,* curd, mashed potato and *moong dal* soup are some Indian foods suitable for diarrhoea patient. Fried food, vegetables, fruits (except banana), milk and milk preparations (except curd and *Matha*) should be avoided during diarrhoea.

ORAL REHYDRATION SOLUTION (ORS)

The fluid and salts lost in watery stools of diarrhoea can be replenished by oral rehydration solution. The formula of the powder of ORS has been arrived at by world Health Organization after years of scientific studies and research. The ORS provides water, glucose, sodium, potassium, chloride and zinc in the same proportion as these are lost in stool. Prompt use of oral rehydration solution has saved millions of precious young lives, threatened by epidemics of diarrhoea and cholera in the third world, bestowing it with coveted name of JEEVAN RAKSHAK GHOL (Life Saving Solution).

One important point to remember is that ORS solution should be prepared strictly according to the instructions given on its wrapper. It should be dissolved in proper amount of water otherwise the altered composition of solution may not be very beneficial and may occasionally harm the user by changing the electrolyte pattern in the blood.

If sachets of ORS powder are not available, a solution of similar quality and efficacy can be made at home with the following composition:-

Water (Boiled & Cooled)	-	1 Glass	200ml.
Sugar (Sucrose)	-	1 Tablespoonful	5gm.
Common Salt (Sodium Chloride)	-	half Teaspoonful	2gm.
Baking Soda (Sodium Bicarbonate)	-	Small Quantity	1gm.
Lemon Juice (Citrate)	-	Few Drops	

If a person having diarrhoea is vomiting or has tendency for vomiting (Nausea) he may require administration of fluid through intravenous route, for which hospitalization may be needed.

Medicines which stop motion by reducing movement of the gut (Anti-motility drugs) should be taken only on the advice of doctor. These medicines may occasionally harm the affected person. We should not forget that frequent loose stool in most cases is an attempt by the body to get rid of harmful and poisonous substances present in the gut.

TRAVELLER'S DIARRHOEA

When citizens of developed nations like USA, Canada, Europe and Australia travel to the developing countries in Asia and Africa, they suffer from episodes of diarrhoea, called traveller's diarrhoea or popularly 'Turista'. Many nick names are given to this condition, like Delhi belly, Hong Kong dog and Kathmandu Quicksteps, highlighting places where it commonly occurs. People travelling the other way like from

India, Nepal and Hong Kong may also get it when they visit United States.

The travellers' diarrhoea is not restricted to international travels. It may happen during inland travel also, if adequate care of hygiene of water and food is not taken.

The most common cause of traveller's diarrhea is infection and release of toxin by Coliform bacteria - Escherichia coli. E coli is present normally in the small intestine, however people from different geographically location harbor different strains of E. coli in their gut. The exposure to new strains of E. coli, carried via food and water may lead to diarrhoea. Apart from the bacteria, many other organisms, like viruses, Giardia, Entamoeba and Worms may also cause diarrhea in a tourist.

Majority of the episodes of traveller's diarrhoea are self limiting. Over a period of 1-2 days the bouts of watery stools cease. In true sense, the formation of watery stool is an attempt by the body to get rid of the new harmful strain of bacteria.

The people visiting South East Asian countries like Thailand and Malaysia, where sea-foods, fish, shrimp and turtle are abundantly consumed, become frequent victims of travellers' diarrhoea.

Persons suffering from this condition rapidly lose water and electrolytes from the body. The treatment therefore is to drink plenty of water to avoid dehydration. A better way to avoid dehydration is to drink Oral Rehydration Solution (ORS) which replenishes the lost salts from the body.

While travelling one should cautiously ensure the cleanliness and freshness of water and food. As far as practicable well cooked, warm food should be eaten and raw salads and fruits should be avoided unless its hygienic standard is quite high.

Roadside food should be avoided and one should visit standard restaurants during travel. If the food served appears to be stale by its flavor and taste, it should be discarded without bothering for the costs involved. The cost of an episode of diarrhoea will be greater than the cost of unhygienic food, thrown away.

It is generally safe to consume biscuits, tea and ripe banana which can be peeled. Bottled and tetra packed fruit juices may safely be taken after checking the date of expiry. Cola drinks and orange juice are acidic and keep the level of E. coli bacteria down.

Curd (*Dahi,* Yogurt) has been proven very effective in bringing back the gut flora to normalcy. It contains a beneficial bacterium - Lactobacillus which checks the growth of harmful bacteria E. coli. One should take curd, prior to and during journey, whenever possible.

CHAPTER-5

• JAUNDICE

Jaundice is yellow discoloration of the skin, nails, eyes and the under surface of the tongue. The normal colour of the urine is pale yellow. It changes to deep yellow similar to that of mustard oil in a patient of jaundice. The change in the colour of skin and urine etc is due to presence of excessive quantity of bile pigments bilirubin.

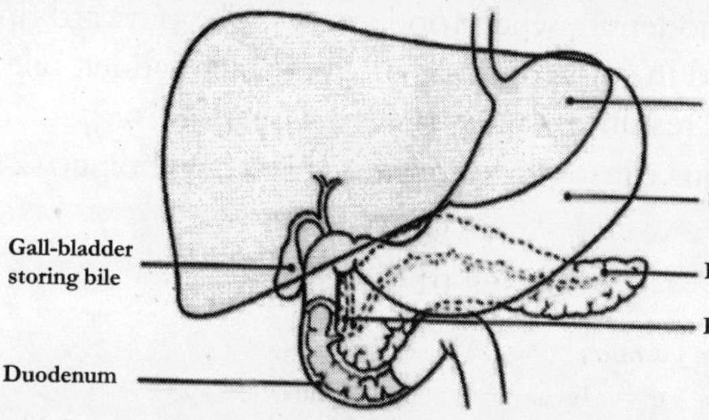

Fig.-7 : Hepato - biliary system

Functions of Liver - Liver, an organ weighing approx 1,500gms in an adult is located in right upper part of the abdomen. Its main job is to filter the blood coming through the portal vein from the intestines. The intestine absorbs the digested food hence the blood sent to liver contains large amount of nutrients. However, this blood also contains small quantity of harmful chemicals. Liver assimilates useful chemicals and stores them. The harmful chemicals and micro organisms are filtered and destroyed. The main functions of liver thus can be enumerated:

1. To assimilate useful molecules like glucose, fat, amino acids and participate in metabolism.
2. To destroy harmful chemicals like ammonia and convert it to urea, which pass out through urine.
3. To help maintain the level of various hormones in blood.
4. To synthesise immune products to fight diseases. It also synthesises albumin and coagulation factors.
5. Storage of Iron, Copper, Vitamin A, D and B12.

Jaundice is only a symptom, caused by various diseases related to blood, liver and biliary system. Bilirubin is the yellow pigment produced by destruction of hemoglobin present in red blood cells. When the production of bilirubin is high due to excessive destruction of red-blood cells (Hemolytic) or when the liver is unable to metabolize it (Hepatocellular) the level of bilirubin rises in blood and jaundice occurs.

The bile produced in liver is stored in gall bladder and released in duodenum when food arrives. The outward flow of bile is blocked in some diseases of liver, gall bladder, bile duct and pancreas resulting in obstructive jaundice.

Various causes of jaundice are listed in box no.-2

Box-2

Causes of Jaundice

A. Hemolytic Jaundice

- Due to excessive breakdown of red blood cells.
- Usually associated with anaemia (Low level of haemoglobin in blood).
- May occur at the time of birth as normal phenomenon, as fetal pattern hemoglobin is replaced by adult pattern.

B. Hepatocellular Jaundice

- Edema and injury to liver due to various reasons:
  1. Virus
  2. Alcohol
  3. Drug Induced
  4. Genetic Defect-metabolic defects

C. Obstructive Jaundice

- Bile is unable to flow out duodenum
  1. Stone in bile duct.
  2. Tumor in the gall bladder, bile duct and pancreas, duodenum
  3. Nodes around bile duct etc.

HEPATITIS

Inflammation or swelling of the liver is termed as Hepatitis. A variety of substances like alcohol, some medicines and organisms may cause swelling of the liver. The hepatitis caused by hepatitis 'B' virus has spread worldwide including India. In this country about 4 crore people are estimated to be infected by hepatitis 'B' virus.

The knowledge about various viruses causing hepatitis has evolved during later part of the last century. The viruses causing hepatitis discovered were named A, B. C etc in sequence of their discovery and gradually their characteristics, mode of spread and virulence were defined. As hepatitis D virus does not have independent existence, at present four important types of hepatitis viruses exist - A, B, C & E. Out of these hepatitis 'A' & 'E' viruses spread through water and food, whereas 'B' & 'C' pass from one person to another via blood , blood products and body fluids.

Hepatitis 'A' & 'E'

The viruses of these two types of hepatitis spread via contaminated water, milk, food and shellfish etc. Infected persons excrete viruses in the faeces which spread to food under poor sanitary conditions. This type of spread of infection is termed Faeco-oral transmission. Outbreaks of Hepatitis 'E' infection has been reported from various parts of North India.

Hepatitis 'A' & 'E' viruses are less dangerous compared to 'B' & 'C' and these generally do not cause long term (chronic) infection. However, acute liver failure is reported in Hepatitis A and E.

Vaccine for prevention of hepatitis 'A' is available, but not for hepatitis 'E'.

Hepatitis 'B' & 'C'

Blood and blood products are the main sources of infection in hepatitis 'B' and 'C'. These viruses may also be present in saliva and tear of an infected person.

The hepatitis 'B' & 'C' infection spreads by contaminated needles, syringes and administration of infected blood products. Transmission of viruses through sexual contact and mother to newborn baby is possible mainly in hepatitis 'B' infection. Surgery, dental treatment and shaving with shared razors and blades are other situations when hepatitis 'B' virus may be transmitted.

The baby of an infected mother generally gets the virus at the time of delivery. If viral load is high in mother, breast feeding may also spread the virus to fetus especially when nipples have cracks, where it gets absorbed through mucosal surface of the fetal gut. Unprotected sex and promiscuity are important factors in hepatitis 'B' transmission and at times in Hepatitis C also.

Hepatitis 'B' infection does not spread by skin contact such as handshaking, hugging and kissing and through droplet infection like sneezing and coughing.

BOX-3

Cause of Hepatitis (Inflammation of Liver)

1. Virus

- Viruses generally harming liver alone are hepatitis 'A', 'B', 'C', and 'E' virus.
- Viruses affecting liver as well as other organs - yellow fever virus, cytomegalo virus etc.

2. Alcohol

- Beer, wine, whisky etc.

3. Medicines

- Anti-tuberculosis drugs like Rifampicin, Isoniazid, Pyrazinamide etc.
- Some Antibiotics like Erythromycine.

Effects of Hepatitis 'B' & 'C'

Majority of the adults (upto 95%) become free of hepatitis 'B' virus infections over a period of 6 months to one year. About five percent persons become long term sufferers and disease goes to the stages of chronic hepatitis and subsequently to liver cirrhosis.

The hepatitis 'B' infection is more stubborn in newborn and children and about 90% of them go to carrier stage, where virus in active or inactive form stays in the baby for more than 6 months.

BOX-4

Precaution to avoid Hepatitis 'B' & 'C' Infection

- Always use disposable syringes and needles. Destroy them after use.
- Do not share shaving razor and tooth brush with anyone.
- Avoid piercing of ear lobes and noses of daughter. If very essential get the services of a qualified surgeon.
- Avoid Tattooing. To be allowed by sterlised needle.
- Avoid promiscuity. Be faithful to spouse. Condom may reduce the risk but can not give guaranteed protection.
- If blood or blood product is to be received ensure their screening for Hepatitis 'B' and other infections.
- Get vaccinated against Hepatitis 'B'. In special situations the success of the vaccine is to be tested when someone in family has hepatitis B infection, with help of some blood tasts.

BEWARE OF HEPATITIS

Probability of your contracting hepatitis increases:

- If there is a patient of hepatitis in your household.
- If your spouse has suffered hepatitis 'B' or 'C'.
- If you are having long standing low grade fever.
- If you are losing weight.
- If glass syringe has been used to give injectible medicines to you, any time in life.
- If you have received blood purchased from market.
- If the result of liver function test (SGOT, SGPT) is found to be abnormal during routine health checkup.
- If you are undergoing or have undergone dialysis.

- You have undergone surgery or tooth extraction.
- If you have suffered from jaundice in past.
- If you are having multiple sexual partners.
- If you belong to high risk group (like Doctors, laboratory staff and Nurses) and have not been vaccinated.

SYMPTOMS OF HEPATITIS

Symptoms of all types of hepatitis are more or less similar and non-specific. The affected person presents with features of acute infectious diseases, such as weakness, malaise, headache, exhaustion and chills. There may be low grade fever, loss of taste and loss of appetite. Associated nausea, vomiting, diarrhoea and upper abdominal pain is common.

Gradually, depending upon the pace of disease, the sclera (white portion of eyes), skin, nails and undersurface of the tongue get discolored yellow, The urine becomes high yellow colored and stool generally acquires a pale hue. Some persons may suffer skin rashes and joint pains.

Majority of the patients of hepatitis recover over a period to 4-8 weeks. In some patients the edema of the liver continues to sub-acute and chronic stages in time frame. Occasional patients undergo severe liver damage leading to acute liver failure.

TREATMENT

Treatment of hepatitis is the domain of the doctor, however following points need proper emphasis:-

A. Any type of self medication or use of unproven medicines, whether it belongs to Allopathy, Ayurvedic or Homeopathy system may prove harmful. Do not make yourself a guinea pig-a subject for experimentation.

B. Rest as advised by the doctor is treatment in hepatitis and also in other viral infections. Take this advice seriously.

C. Take nutritious diet including good amount of glucose, fruit drinks and also protein. Many patients of hepatitis are literally starved due to superstitious beliefs of their attendants.

D. The administration of now available antiviral medicines is guided by duration of hepatitis, viral load and the degree of on-going effects on the liver. A proper decision to give antiviral drugs and its dose etc can only be taken by a qualified physician or a hepatologist.

PREVENTION

Apart from taking precautions to avoid hepatitis (Box no.-4), one should take a course of vaccine to prevent hepatitis. At present immune serum globulin and vaccines are available for hepatitis 'A' & 'B'.

(1) Immune Serum Globulin - It provides immediate protection from the specific infection, however its effects lasts for a short time only. This is called passive immunisation as the immune product is supplied from outside.

Babies born of Hepatitis 'B' positive mothers are at high risk of contracting it. They should be given immunoglobulin against hepatitis 'B' within 12 hours of birth.

(2) Vaccination - The injections of vaccines stimulate the body to produce its own immunoglobulin against a particular disease. This immunity lasts longer, is more effective and is called active immunization. Generally three injections at defined timing are given for hepatitis 'B' vaccination.

Now days it has become essential to check hepatitis 'B' status (by testing blood for hepatitis 'B' surface antigen) before giving the course of vaccine in adults, otherwise if the person is already carrying the hepatitis B virus he would not benefit from the vaccination and later may blame the vaccine if he/she will develop features of hepatitis.

Children are exempt from this mandate, provided there is no history of jaundice in the child and his family in the past.

CONTACT WITH HEPATITIS PATIENTS

Viral Hepatitis does not spread by simple physical contact like touching, shaking hand, hugging or kissing. Sharing room, bed, sofa or toilet also does not spread it.

The transmission of hepatitis 'A' and 'E' is faeco-oral i.e. through contaminated water and food. A person having these types of hepatitis should thoroughly wash hands after every visit to toilet and before cooking food.

Hepatitis 'B' & 'C' may communicate by intimate physical and sexual contact.

DIET AND REST IN HEPATITIS

Generally the patients of jaundice are given only bland and boiled food. Bland taste of such foods along with loss of appetite due to disease, leads to undernourishment and patients gradually become weak. It is wrong to think that yellow colored foods; pulses, turmeric and mango etc contribute to jaundice.

A patient of jaundice should be given hygienic, palatable and easily digestible foods, similar to what other members of a household partake. There is no need to cook separately for a jaundiced patient. Small quantity of fat in the form of cooking oil and butter may also be given, though very fatty and fried food like *paratha,* pizza, milk cream etc should be avoided.

Fruit and fruit juices are safe and provide various vitamins. Fibre content of fruit stimulates bowel movement and prevents constipation. Utmost hygienic care is essential, while extracting fruit juice to avoid infection and subsequent diarrhoea. Coconut water and packed fruit juices are generally safe. Non-vegetarian food, as it is more difficult to digest should preferably be avoided in jaundice

Salt

Patients of jaundice should be given food with normal salt content. Low salt diet may lead to overall low intake of food and undernourishment.

Patients of jaundice who develop edema and ascites (collection of fluid in the peritoneal cavity) may be advised low salt diet by the doctor.

Rest

Patients of jaundice are advised rest which is an integral part of the treatment. Bed rest reduces the demand of glucose produced by the liver as well as it improves the flow of blood to liver.

The mental work does not consume much energy. There is no restriction in studying and doing paper and office work. Teaching at home should be arranged for children having jaundice.

Physical activities like running and outdoor sports should not be performed by a jaundice patient. These hectic physical activities may drastically reduce blood sugar level leading to exhausion and serious consequences.

Jaundiced patient employed in jobs demanding hard physical labour may require discontinuing job temporarily.

Hepatitis 'B' and Pregnancy

Pregnant women are now routinely screened for hepatitis 'B' infection during antenatal check up. When the mother is found to be negative she is given full course of hepatitis 'B' vaccination without waiting for delivery of the child.

When the mother is found positive for hepatitis 'B' surface antigen the probability of baby contracting it is quite high. This mother to child passage of infection is called vertical transmission.

Mothers with hepatitis 'B' infection have increased risk of abortion and of delivery before due time (Preterm delivery).

The doctor has to take care of two individuals - mother and the baby, in such situations.

Hepatitis 'B' infected mother is investigated for its effect on liver. Quantitative assessment of viral load is done and treatment is given according to the results of the investigations. Antiviral medicines may be given to pregnant mother to reduce, Mother to Child, transmission of hepatitis 'B' infection during labour.

CARE OF THE NEWBORN BABY

New born baby of hepatitis 'B' positive mother should be given immunoglobulin (Passive Immunisation) as well as vaccine (Active Immunisation) within 12 hours of birth.

Breast-feeding by hepatitis 'B' positive mother

Breastfeeding is allowed if the child is vaccinated and the mother is not taking antiviral medications. The child ingests viruses present in the breast milk and in the blood if the mother has cracked nipples. Nipple shield may be used to cover the cracks and minimize the possibility of infection. Opinion of an expert for breastfeeding should be sought if the mother is taking antiviral medicines.

Child-bearing during antiviral therapy for Hepatitis B & C infections

Hepatitis B & C positive women should be treated by suitable medicines, before they plan child bearing. Pregnancy should preferably be avoided during this antiviral treatment.

CHAPTER- 6

• OBESITY

Physical activity is essential to keep a human body fit and healthy. The predecessors of modern man lived in the forests along with wild animals, where staying physically strong was must for survival. Therefore the genetic configuration of human body is designed for physical activity.

The weight of a healthy person should be within a range depending upon age, sex, height and race. A person having greater than recommended weight, is termed overweight or obese.

If the weight is 10 to 20 percent above the desirable weight, it is called overweight. When the weight is 20% or more above the maximum desirable weight it is labelled obesity.

Sedentary life style and overeating are two main factors that lead to obesity. An obese person is prone to have many diseases like Hypertension, Diabetes and Coronary Artery Disease. Physical activities like walking, jogging, swimming and playing football, hockey, badminton etc. stimulate intestine, propel food and let the wind pass. Large amount of energy is spent in physical activity, whereas minimal calorie is consumed by mental work. Physical activities relieve constipation and improve appetite.

About five crore people out of present Indian population of approx 120 crores are obese. In urban areas of few northern states like Delhi, Punjab, Rajasthan and Gujarat about 30% of adult population is obese. Uncontrolled eating of fatty foods has led to high incidence of obesity even in middle and lower middle socio economic groups. In India people enjoy 'fatty food' rather than 'healthy food'. Food for many persons is recreation and at psychological level they **'live for eating'** rather than **'eat for living'**, leading to obesity.

In many Indian households the overall use of fat (*Ghee,* Oil, and Butter etc) is quite high. Festivals and celebrations of child birth and marriage etc offer added opportunities to overeat.

Women of child bearing age group gain weight during every pregnancy, which they generally do not shed after the birth of the child and this way after two or three pregnancies women become overweight.

In some persons stress and depression contribute to obesity as they find solace and pleasure in eating.

DEGREE OF OBESITY

In order to estimate the degree of obesity doctors calculate the 'Body-Mass Index' (BMI), according to the formula:-

Body Mass Index = (weight in kg.) ÷ (Height in meter)^2

BMI - up to 25 - Normal

25-29.9 - Overweight

30 and above 30 - Obese.

Obesity increases the risk of many diseases; however the risk also depends upon the pattern of obesity.

1. ABDOMINAL OBESITY (TRUNCAL OBESITY) - In this situation fat is deposited mainly over abdomen (tummy) and the shape of trunk becomes similar to the shape of apple.

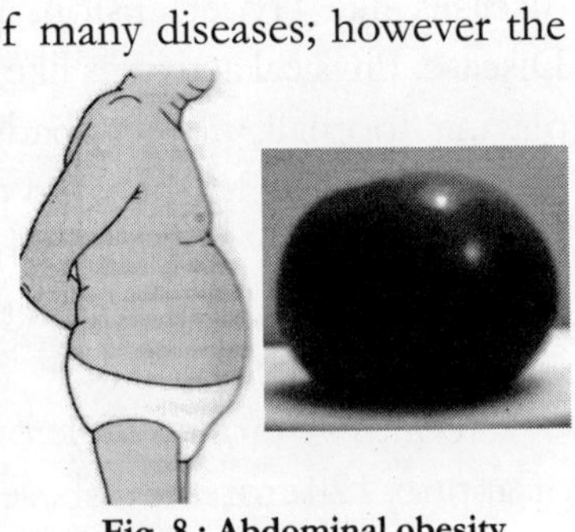

Fig.-8 : Abdominal obesity (Apple shape)

Such persons are at greater risk of having hypertension and coronary artery disease.

2. GENERALISED OBESITY - In this pattern fat is distributed all over the body and more fat is deposited over the hip compared to the waist. The shape of trunk of such person becomes comparable to the outline of a pear. Generalised obesity is less risky compared to abdominal obesity.

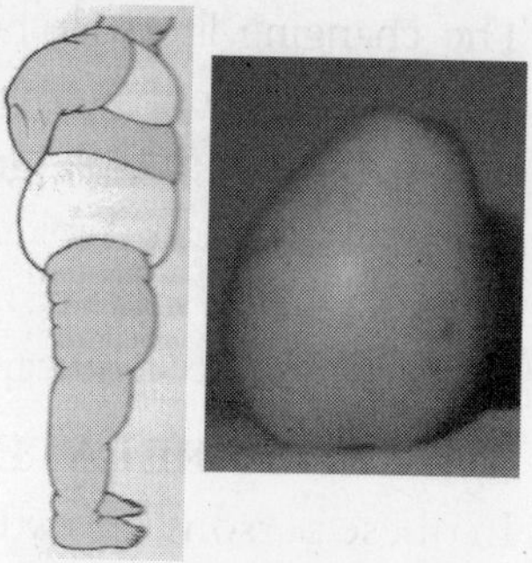

Fig.-9 : Generalized obesity (Pear shape)

These two patterns of body fat distribution may be differentiated by calculating "Waist to Hip Ratio". To find this ratio the measurement of circumference of waist (at the level of umbilicus) is divided by the circumference of hip (at the level of buttocks). A ratio, more than 1.0 in males and 0.8 in females is associated with greater chances of ischemic heart disease.

An absolute value of waist circumference of more than 80cms is also considered abnormal in adults of any height, age or sex.

FACTORS UNDERLYING OBESITY

Irrespective of the contribution of life style and overeating, some people tend to become obese.

Hereditary - Some persons are genetically prone to become obese. Obesity runs in their families and majority of members are affected by it.

Diseases - The deficiency of thyroid hormone (Hypothyroidism) is a frequent cause of obesity. Women undergoing surgical removal of uterus also many a times gain weight due to changes in the hormonal profile of the body. These situations need attention and analysis by a specialist doctor.

The changing life style however is the major reason for rising incidence of obesity in our population. In urban areas the paucity of open spaces and playgrounds compels people to stay indoors, watching television. Avoiding walking, using lifts instead of staircare and going even short distances by car or scooter, though appear trivial contribute significantly to weight gain.

AILMENTS RELATED TO OBESITY

In obese persons the extra fat is deposited underneath skin and also at the interfaces of the organs in the abdomen. Apart from these, the fat content of the liver is increased (Fatty liver), that interferes with proper working of liver and may cause jaundice.

The fat deposits in the inner lining of blood vessels forming elevated patches-plaques. This condition, known as Atherosclerosis, makes the blood vessel lose its elasticity and leads to high blood pressure, coronary artery disease, heart-attack and brain-stroke.

Compared to average population an obese person has more chances to suffer gall bladder stone, hernia, joint pains, fungal infection, diabetes and kidney diseases.

TREATMENT

While trying to reduce weight one has to firmly believe that the obesity is a disease. When someone is convinced with the dictum, then only a sincere effort at weight reduction can be made. A strong will-power and consistent effort to reduce weight and keep it low is required as any slackness may lead to regain in the weight.

The first and foremost thing is a medical consultation to exclude any underlying reason for obesity, assess associated problems (diabetes, high blood pressure) and their bad effect on target organs–eyes, kidneys, feet, nerves, brain and heart etc. Under medical supervision, the reduction in calorie intake and increase in energy expenditure will lead to reduction in weight (See Box no.-5).

Some anti-obesity medicines are also available these days which may be taken on prescription by a qualified physician. In extreme cases of obesity, bariatric surgery may be advised. In this surgery the size of the stomach is reduced by stapling or removing part of it and the person gets a feel of full tummy or satiety even with small quantity of food.

BOX-5

Ways to Reduce Weight

A. Time and Place of Eating

- Eat at fixed time and place. This way continuous munching leading to excessive food intake may be avoided.
- Eat slowly, relaxingly, chewing every bolus of food at least 15-20 times. You will feel satiety with lesser quantity of food.
- Concentrate on food while eating. Do not watch television, read book or indulge in serious discussion while eating.
- Take food in company of persons who eat frugally or in normal quantity. Avoid company of people dedicated to food.(Over eaters)
- Serve food in small plates and bowls. Even small quantity of food will give impression of the plate being full.
- Eat slightly less than your hunger. You will feel better with light tummy.

B. Type of Food

- Have plenty of green leafy vegetables and salad in your food. Tomato, Carrot, Reddish and Cucumber etc have low calorie content.
- Take salads and cooked vegetables first to fill the tummy, then relish small quantities of cereals.
- Avoid fatty food, like fried rice, *paratha, puree* and sweets. Do not even keep these things on dining table as you may eat out of impulse.
- The best Indian sweet containing minimum fat is white *Rosogulla.* Other sweets like *Gulabjamun, Bundi ka laddoo, sonpapri* etc have heavy quantity of fat.
- Reduce overall consumption of fat and cooking oil in your household.
- Take a few glasses of water 15-20 minutes before eating.

C. Fasting

- Fasting, as it is generally followed by overeating does not help in weight reduction.

D. Exercise

- Physical activity, exercise and outdoor games are must for healthy living. Walking, jogging, cycling, playing football etc make you physically strong. These activities burn calorie, improve appetite and may increases food allowance.
- Exhaustion out of physical activity leads to better sleep.

CHAPTER- 7

WATER AND WATER BORN DISEASES

Water is a key constituent of our body. The adult human body has 60% and an infant's body has 75% content as water. Water content of various fluids of the body; blood, digestive juice, saliva, mother's milk and urine is more than 90%

We ingest water in the form of milk, soup, fruit juices and plain water etc. The water is shed out of body in exhaled air, urine, stool and sweat. Our kidneys maintain the balance of water content of body by varying the quantity of urine.

Most of the nutrients; amino acids, glucose, vitamins and minerals are soluble in water. These biological chemicals need water molecules to enter and exit cells. Water is essential to maintain the turgidity of cells to facilitate metabolic activities.

The overall requirement of water depends upon the age of the person, temperature and humidity of the surrounding, physical activity and other factors like pregnancy. An adult takes about 2-4 liters of water every day including the amount ingested with food.

Vomiting, diarrhoea, excessive perspiration and low intake of water reduce the water content of body leading to dehydration. More than 20 percent reduction in water content of the body may be hazardous. Thirst is a signal indicating reduced water content in the body.

Excess of water causes swelling of feet and puffiness of the face. Excessive fluid retention may lead to abnormal fluid collection in abdomen (Ascites), Chest (Pleural Effusion) and around heart (Pericardial Effusion).

Water aids as a medium for absorption of nutrients in the intestine. Impure and contaminated water may allow entry of harmful organisms and chemicals through the intestinal mucosa. The absorption of food, medicines as well as poison depends upon water. A large number of abdominal problems are caused by taking contaminated water:

BOX-6

WATER BORN INFECTIOUS DISEASES

A. Protozoa – Diarrhoea (Amoebiasis, Giardiasis).

B. Bacteria - Dysentry (Shigella), Enteric Fever (Salmonella), Cholera (Vibrio cholerae).

C. Virus - Viral diarrhoea, Poliomyelitis, Hepatitis 'A' and 'E'.

D. Worms - Round worm (Ascariasis), Thread worm (Enterobiasis), Hook worm (Ankylostomiasis), Tape worm (Taenia solium and saginata).

PROTOZOA

Amoebiasis and Giardiasis cause diarrhoea, by interfering with the digestion of food and absorption of the water. The infected person passes frequent watery stool.

BACTERIA

In Bacterial dysentery, small quantities of stool mixed with blood and mucus are passed intermittently.

Cholera is caused by the bacteria Vibrio cholerae. The victim gets recurrent attacks of rice water like stool along with vomiting. Rapidly setting dehydration due to fluid loss, threatens the life of victim.

VIRUS

Viruses may also cause diarrhoea. A child infected with polio virus, may initially suffer from diarrhoea. Viral hepatitis type 'A' & 'E' spread through contaminated water.

WORMS IN INTESTINE

Varieties of worms enter our gastrointestinal tract through contaminated water and food and reside in the inner lining of mucosa. The worms grow at the expense of the host, stealing the nutrients from the intestinal mucosa. Following are the main types of worms found in human intestines:-

1. Round Worm (Ascaris)
2. Thread Worm (Enterobiasis)
3. Hook Worm (Ancylostomiasis)
4. Tape Worm (Taenia solium & T. saginata)
5. Others - Whip worm, T.trichura etc.

1. Round Worm (Ascaris)

This yellowish, 20-35cm long worm resembles earthworm and spreads by eating food contaminated with its egg. Ascaris may cause pain abdomen, malnourishment and obstruction in the intestines. They may migrate to bile duct causing biliary colic, jaundice and Pancreatitis.

Adult worms can be expelled rectally or orally. Occasionally, the worms are demonstrated in barium examination of gut as linear filling defects.

Its larva passes through lungs during its life cycle in human beings, when it may cause cough, breathlessness and eosinophilia.

Ascaris is the most prevalent worm infestation and community treatment programme are recommended to lower its prevalence.

2. THREAD WORM (Enterobiasis)

These thread like, upto 1.5cm long, white worms are commonly seen around the anus of children. The worms may be seen on the buttock and in the faeces. It causes intense itching, around anus.

The eggs of the thread worm dropped around anus are picked up in nails during scratching and re-enter the body during finger-sucking and eating with unwashed fingers.

The cycle of re-infection may continue for long periods in absence of treatment. The cycle may be interrupted by following measures:

1. Keep the fingernails short.
2. Thoroughly clean hands including nails before meals.
3. Clothe children in undergarments with elastic bands at waist and thigh. Anal scratching with cloth covering will not let the eggs pass in finger nails.
4. Treat all children in a family or hostel simultaneously.

3. HOOK WORM (Ancylostomiasis)

The adult hook worm is up to 1 cm long and resides in the duodenum. It sucks blood and causes anemia.

The entry and path of the hookworm in human body is quite peculiar. Eggs passed in the faeces develop into larvae in moist soil; they then penetrate human skin and reach lungs via blood vessels. From lungs they travel to bronchi and enter digestive tract on swallowing, finally making duodenum their final habitat.

The larvae entering the skin of foot may cause local swelling and redness. While in lung it may cause cough, breathlessness and eosinophilia. When the hook worms are in gut, abdominal pain, vomiting and loose stool occurs.

Hook worm infection may cause undernourishment, anaemia and low protein levels in blood. Heavy worm load in children may lead to physical and mental growth retardation, and in adults it may cause severe anaemia which may lead to heart failure.

4. Tape Worm (Taenia solium and Taenia saginata)

These long, segmented ribbon shaped worms inhabit small intestine. The square shaped broken segments passed in faeces resemble pumpkin seeds.

Infection is caused by eating improperly cooked contaminated pork (T. Solium) or beef (T. Saginata). The transmission of tapeworm is faeco-oral.

The adult worm resides in intestine, where as the larvae penetrate the intestinal mucosa and are carried to many parts of body where they form cysts (Cysticercosis). Cysts placed under skin and in muscles may be palpable as pea size ovoid bodies. Cysts of Taenia solium in the brain (Neuro cysticercosis) may cause epileptic fits in adults and encephalitis in heavily infected children.

Cooking pork and beef properly will prevent tapeworm infection. Faecal contamination of drinking water, vegetables and foods should be avoided to reduce overall prevalence of tapeworm infection in community.

Prevention of water born infections

Water born infections spread by drinking contaminated water and infected raw, uncooked foods.

Clean Potable Water

One must ensure the drinking water is free from infective organisms. The rural practice of defeacating in open and washing in river bed and pond water should be stopped to prevent faeco-oral spread of infections.

The water may get infected at source, during supply and at the site of storage. The quality of water of deep tube wells is generally good as it is drawn from below the layers of rock. Unfortunately due to heavy pollution the water table has also become contaminated at many places. The supply pipes in many areas are old, corroded and laid along the drainage system. The water passing in these pipes may suck impurities from outside.

Where ever possible water should be cleaned by filter, aquaguard or R.O. System. Clean potable water should be arranged in schools, clinics, offices, railway stations and other public places.

Uncooked Food

Uncooked food materials; salads, fruits, chutney are good source of micro-organisms and spores of worms. Vegetables including palak, raddish, coriander leaves should be thoroughly cleaned before eating. Fruit salads and fruit juices from roadside vendors should be avoided.

CHAPTER-8

• HYPERACIDITY AND GAS

A. Dyspepsia & Heartburn

Dyspepsia refers to the discomfort caused by bloating of abdomen with gas associated with burping and nausea. It is a non-specific symptom and may arise due to overeating or consuming stale or improperly cooked food. Dyspepsia may occasionally be due to some serious underlying disease of the stomach, gall bladder, pancreas and intestine - the organs which secrete digestive juices.

Many patients of dyspepsia also suffer from heartburn, a burning pain in the upper abdomen and behind the breast bone (sternum), caused by the passage of gastric acid to the esophagus. The digestive juice secreted in stomach is acidic in nature and under normal circumstances it flows forwards towards duodenum and small intestine. It's backward flow and entry into esophagus is blocked by a valve like mechanism at its junction with the stomach. The deficient working of the valve at gastro-esophageal junction and the motility disorders of stomach and small intestine cause reflux of acid and heartburn.

Cold water, cold drink, ice-cream, fast food and alcohol may cause gastro esophageal reflux, hyperacidity and dyspepsia. Fatty food, chocolate and peppermint may also produce similar effect.

The refluxing acid may cause cough and induce an attack of asthma in susceptible persons. Long standing reflux of acid, reaching upto throat and mouth may cause hoarseness of voice and discoloration of the teeth. Measures to avoid gastro esophageal reflux and heartburn are listed in Box no.-7

Patients of dyspepsia and heartburn require upper gastro intestinal endoscopy examination to exclude ulcer, stricture and cancer in upper gastrointestinal Tract. The symptoms of simple hyperacidity as well as those arising out of cancerous ulcer in the stomach are similar and initially equally be improved with the use of antacid and other acid reducing measures.

BOX-7

Measures to Avoid Hyperacidity and Heartburn

A. To Avoid Hyperacidity

- Reduce intake of tea, coffee and aerated beverages. Stop alcohol and smoking.
- Reduce intake of fatty and deep fried food.
- Avoid non-vegetarian foods-meat, fish and eggs.
- Reduce intake of *Papad,* Pickles.
- Avoid citrus fruits-orange, *mausambi.* Squeeze lemon juice in some food item like *dal* and *sabzi* (Pulses and vegetables)
- Avoid pain-relieving medicines like aspirin, ibuprofen, diclofenac etc.

B. To Avoid gastro esophageal reflux

- Do not take large quantity of food at one sitting. Keeping the overall intake of food constant spread it over five times instead of three times a day.
- Reduce weight, if you are overweight.
- Take light meal in the evening and night. Take super at least two hours before going to bed.
- Walk for 15 minutes leisurely over level ground after the supper.
- Do not wear tight trouser and belt.
- If the reflux is severe elevate the head end of the bed by putting a brick (6"high) under its legs.

B. Peptic Ulcer

An ulcer in the inner lining of stomach or duodenum is called peptic ulcer. Increase in the amount of gastric acid or poor healing power is thought to be underlying cause of peptic ulcer, however at present the bacteria 'Helicobacter Pylori' is considered to be the main culprit. The presence of bacteria in stomach can be ascertained by biochemical test of the tissue taken from stomach with gastroscopy equipment. The bacteria helicobacter generally can be eradicated by a course of specific antibiotics. Serological test in blood can also defect H. Pyloric infection.

In a patient having acidity and gas, the doctor has to judge whether the dominant factor is increase in quantity of gastric acid or the gastro esophageal reflux and prescribe medicines accordingly. A peptic ulcer may bleed causing anemia, melaena (Black stool) and haematemesis (Vomiting of blood).

Avoidance of fatty and spicy food, aerated drinks and alcohol and stopping smoking may relieve symptoms of gas and dyspepsia. The quantity of tea and coffee intake should be cut down. Pain-killer medicines like aspirin, ibuprofen ,nimuselide and diclofenac should be avoided by patients of hyperacidity and peptic ulcer.

C. Abdominal gas

Increase in intestinal gases, causing abdominal distension, rumbling sound in tummy and frequent per-anal passage of gas is a common malady in our population. Presence of gas in the intestine is normal; however undue increase in its quantity is discomforting and socially embarrassing.

While eating, drinking or swallowing, a small quantity of air is also swallowed. Though it sounds weird, every act of swallowing ingests 2-3ml of air, totaling 2-3 liters per day. It is quite natural that this ingested amount of air has to be farted or burped out. Generally the swallowed air containing nitrogen, oxygen and carbon dioxide is odorless.

The process of digestion and fermentation in small intestine also produces small amount of mal-odorous gases like ammonia and hydrogen sulfide. High fibre food, generally considered good for health, causes increase in gas production. Whole wheat bread, legumes, fruits, vegetables, onion and salads contain high amount of fibre and produce more gas due to bacterial action.

Per anal passage of gas, flatulence releases between 500-1500ml of gas every day depending upon the diet and body habits. This is generally more of a social embarrassment than a disease.

D. Aerophagy

Some people voluntarily release the air from stomach (burping or eructation) with a noisy sound and in the process ingest greater quantity of air. Generally such persons are tense and/or depressed. The Aerophagy is commoner in women and may be a deliberate act to draw attention. Psychological evaluation and emotional support may be needed to alleviate it.

The symptoms of gas, heartburn and abdominal bloating are generally harmless, however, when these are associated with vomiting, fever, loss of weight or black stool, the doctor should immediately be consulted as the latter symptoms are indicators of some serious problem.

CHAPTER- 9

DISEASES OF MOUTH AND FOOD PIPE (ESOPHAGUS)

Mouth is the point of entry of food in our body. The bolus of food is chewed and crushed in the mouth. It is mixed here with saliva which lubricates the food and adds digestive enzymes.

The tongue has many taste buds on its surface which make us appreciate the taste of the food and differentiate the salt from sugar and sweet from sour. The tongue along with muscles of cheek and palate move the food forwards towards teeth during chewing and backwards in throat during swallowing and onwards passage to food pipe and stomach.

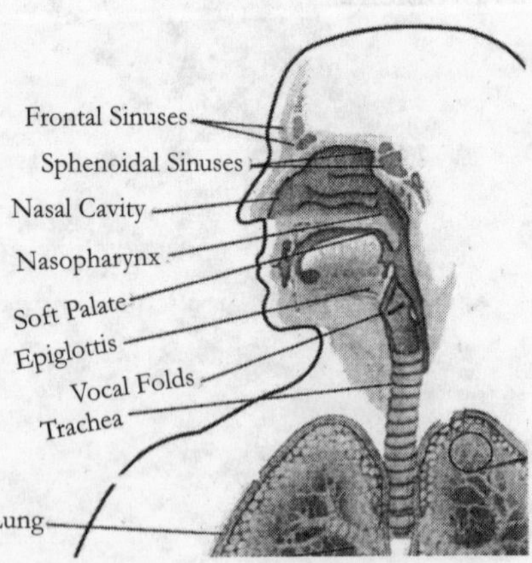

Fig.-10 : Sectional View of Mouth and Throat

Saliva is produced by three sets of salivary glands located around mouth. It moistens the mouth, thereby helping in tasting, chewing, swallowing as well as in digesting the starch present in food. Three pairs of salivary glands; parotid, submandibular and sublingual produce about 1.5 litre of saliva every day.

The main diseases of mouth are bad breath (Halitosis), loss of taste (Dysgeusia), difficulty in swallowing (dysphagia) and hiccup.

BAD BREATH (Halitosis)

Bad breath or unpleasant odour of exhaled air is caused by the growth of bacteria in the mouth and throat. Whenever we take food, milk, tea and juice and do not rinse mouth thoroughly afterwards, a film of food matter settles in mouth, on which micro colonies of bacteria grow. The bacteria produce minute quantities of malodorous gases causing bad breath.

Bad breath is more pronounced when there are pockets of infections in the mouth such as caries teeth, gingivitis and tonsillitis.

One of the functions of saliva is to cleanse the mouth. During sleep the secretion of saliva is reduced causing bad breath in morning even in otherwise normal persons. The quantity of salivary fluid decreases with advancing age. Smoking reduces salivation and makes the tongue hairy, where food particles are trapped facilitating the bacterial overgrowth. The digestion of garlic and onion produces sulphurous gases causing bad breath.

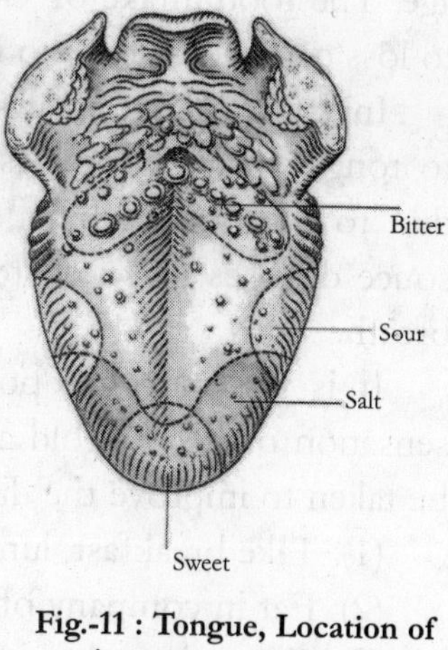

Fig.-11 : Tongue, Location of various types of taste buds

Tartar, the yellow crust like deposit on teeth helps bacteria grow. One must regularly get the services of a dentist to remove tartar. Removal of tartar strengthens teeth by allowing better grip of gums on the teeth.

Citrus fruits like orange, lemon, amla etc contain good amount of vitamin C (Ascorbic Acid). These along with tomato and green leafy vegetables should be regularly taken to keep gums and teeth healthy.

Loss of Taste (Ageusia)

The appreciation of taste depends upon the taste buds located on the surface of tongue. The buds for sweet, salty, bitter and sour tastes are located in different parts of the tongue. A person must be able to appreciate tastes of lemon juice (sour), sugar solution (sweet), table salt (salty) and bitter gourd (Bitter).

Adequate quantity of saliva is required for taste perception, as the buds can only appreciate the taste of liquid substances. It is not possible to taste solid and dry foods, until these are dissolved by saliva.

The number and sensitivity of taste buds decreases with age. The food intake of elderly persons may be reduced due to loss of taste, leading to loss of weight and energy.

Injury to head, paralysis and disorders of nerves going to tongue may disturb taste perception. Dryness of mouth due to mouth-breathing, medication (atropine group) and souce diseases may lead to loss of taste and may cause bad breath.

It is generally not possible to improve the diminished sensation of taste in old age; however certain measures may be taken to improve the diet:

(1) Take breakfast, lunch and dinner timely
(2) Eat in company of friends and family members
(3) Take coloured fruits, vegetables. Add sweets in the diet.

Hiccups

Diaphragm is the muscular tissue that separates thoracic cavity (Heart and Lung) and abdominal cavity. It moves down during breathing in and moves up during breathing out.

Hiccup is a discomforting condition when involuntary contraction of the diaphragm causes rush of air in the lungs and sudden termination of process causes a typical hiccup sound.

The diseases of esophagus, diaphragm and stomach may cause hiccup. Eating rapidly or ingestion of large amount of food and aerated drink distends stomach and the air trapped in its upper fundal part may trigger hiccup by pressing the diaphragm.

Many episodes of hiccup are psychic in origin and triggered by emotional stress. Generally hiccup correct spontaneously within a day or two. Persistent hiccup may disturb food intake. Liver and kidney failure and increased intracranial tension may also cause hiccups, warranting medical attention.

Difficulty in Swallowing (Dysphagia)

Inflammation in throat (Pharyngitis) and tonsils (Tonsillitis) may make the act of swallowing difficult and painful. Ulcers on tongue and in the throat may cause dysphagia.

Diseases of aesophagus like esophageal web, ring, inflammation (oesophagitis), diverticula and tumor may cause difficulty in swallowing. Patient may express that food gets arrested at the level of breast bone. Long standing gastro-esophageal reflux may damage esophageal mucosa causing dysphagia.

Some emotionally disturbed persons feel a lump in the throat at the time of eating (Globus hystericus). Patient of dysphagia require endoscopic observation of throat and esophagus to exclude any disease process before declaring it to be harmless.

PRECAUTIONS

- One should avoid taking very hot as well as very cold food and drinks as it may damage the lining of food pipe and may also cause momentary motility disorder.
- Take adequate amount of water while swallowing pills. One or two gulps should be taken initially to moisten the esophagus followed by the tablet and a few more gulps of water to let it reach the stomach. Taking pills without water (especially doxycycline capsule) may cause ulcers in food pipe leading to dysphagia.
- A few sips of water should be taken to clear the esophagus after ingesting liquid medications.

CHAPTER-10

MILK AND LACTOSE INTOLERANCE

Milk is an essential item in our diet. This is a rich source of protein, vitamins, energy and calcium. Calcium gives strength to our bones. Women who are pregnant and breast feeding their babies require greater amount of calcium in the diet.

Vegetarians fulfil their requirement of protein by milk and pulses. Milk is a complete food. It supplies all the components of nutrition except iron and vitamin B12. The excellent growth and development of a newborn child on breast feed proves that milk is a wholesome food. Mother's milk is generally considered ideal food for newborn babies and infants up to one year of age.

Milk for human consumption is generally procured from cows and buffaloes. At some places she-goat, sheep, camel and reindeer are also milked. All these animals belong to mammalian phyllum and produce milk for their own offspring.

The cow's milk is composed of water (87%), fat (3.7%), protein (5%), lactose, minerals and vitamins. The composition of the milk of other animals differs only marginally from it. Milk is a perishable item and remains fit for drinking for longer period when kept in a freeze or stored after boiling. The transportation of milk to long distances requires special refrigerated vessels where it is kept at temperature below 8 degree centigrade.

PASTEURISATION

Pasteurisation is a process which kills bacteria in milk and prevents spread of milk-born pathogens. The process is named after Louis Pasteur, a great scientist who proved that bacteria are present in air. He also unravelled the mystery of fermentation.

PROCESS

In Pasteurisation the milk is heated to 60°C temperature where it is simmered for 30 minutes. Its temperature is then raised to 80°C for few minutes and then rapidly brought down to zero degree. These changes in the temperature of the milk coagulate the protein of bacteria, killing them without altering the protein of milk.

The use of pasteurized milk drastically lowers the incidence of gut infections. Drinking non-pasteurized milk from infected cows may cause tuberculosis of intestines. It is worth mentioning that simple boiling does not achieve the same objective as Pasteurisation, as the two are distinct processes.

It is strongly recommended to consume pasteurized milk where ever it is available. Pasteurised milk should also be boiled before storage and consumption.

RAW MILK

'Drinking raw milk is better for health', is not true. Boiling makes the milk easier to digest and also kills micro-organisms. When the cow herd is infected the probability of contracting infection increases on consuming raw milk, compared to drinking Pasteurised and boiled milk.

The milk supplied by dairy projects has some additional benefits apart from effects of Pasteurization. The composition of the milk is maintained by adding milk solid and milk fat. A variety of milk with different compositions is supplied to suit individual needs:-

1. **Standard Milk -** (Milk fat 4.5%, milk solid 8.5%) It is suitable for children and for general use.
2. **Half toned Milk -** (Milk fat 3%, milk solid 8.5%) It is suitable for overweight adults and children.
3. **Full toned Milk -** (Milk solid 1.5%, milk solid 8.5%). It has low fat content. Good for adding in tea. Full toned milk is recommended for the obese people.

As milk is an important source of calcium and protein the diet of every person should contain milk and milk products equivalent to approximately half a litre of milk.

LACTOSE INTOLERANCE

Some individuals complain of bloating up with gas, intestinal rumblings and abdominal cramps following ingestion of milk. Such persons, said to have lactose intolerance, may also suffer nausea and diarrhoea. This intolerance to milk is due to their inability to digest lactose, a type of sugar present in milk. The small intestines of such persons do not produce enough lactase, the enzyme needed to digest lactose.

Many people develop some degree of lactose intolerance with advancing age. This is not a dangerous or life threatening condition, however it may occasionally be quite discomforting.

Following measure may help in overcoming lactose intolerance:-

1. Take small quantity of milk at a time, such as a cup of milk
2. Take preparation of milk like custard, *kheer, siwai, paneer* and *rasgullah.*
3. Put few tablespoonfuls of horlicks, boost, complan or similar powder in milk.
4. Take milk boiled with a teaspoonful of *saunf.*
5. Take yogurt *(Dahi).* The bacteria lactobacillus present in yogurt produces the enzyme lactase improving its digestion. Lactobacilli also replace the harmful bacteria in the gut, protecting us from gastroenteritis.

Yogurt may either be taken sweetened or with a pinch of salt in it. A variety of tasty preparation can be made with yogurt as base.

It is important to note that yogurt supplied by dairy projects does not give the benefit of lactobacilli, as its repasteurisation inactivates them. To get this benefit one must take fresh home made yogurt.

CHAPTER-11

INVESTIGATION IN ABDOMINAL PROBLEMS

The modern medical science advocates evidence based approach for proper diagnosis and treatment of diseases. When a person suffers from an illness a provisional diagnosis, based upon history of the illness and clinical examination of the body, is made. In order to support the provisional diagnosis and exclude other possibilities; certain tests of urine, stool and blood are performed and images of the organs are taken with the help of Ultrasonography etc. The evidences thus gathered are analysed to get a proper and final diagnosis which help to formulate the line of treatment.

1. URINE TEST

The presence of bile pigments, bile salts and urobilinogen in urine lead to confirmation of jaundice and indicate its possible cause. In the common hepatocellular jaundice the level of urobilinogen in urine is high whereas it is found to be low in cases of obstructive jaundice, where the bile duct is blocked due to stone or tumour.

The presence of sugar in urine suggests diabetes. Excessive quantity of albumin in urine points towards renal disease. The presence of red blood cells in urine of a person having an attack of abdominal pain suggests renal stone to be the probable cause.

2. STOOL TEST

The tests of stool give invaluable information in the abdominal problems. The cysts and active forms of harmful amoeba (Entamoeba histolytica) and eggs of various worms can be seen by microscopic examination of stool. The eggs of round worm, thread worm, hook worm and tape worm etc. have distinctive appearance under the lens of the microscope.

When there is large amount of bleeding in the gastrointestinal tract it is seen either as fresh red blood or altered tarry black stool. Minute amounts of blood in the stool can be detected by testing for 'Occult blood' by special techniques. This may help in finding the cause of anemia and suggest presence of ulcers, tumors in stomach and other parts of gut where from the blood has oozed slowly and caused anemia.

3. BLOOD TEST

The level of Hemoglobin, number of red and white blood cells and measurements of various enzymes like SGPT and SGOT in blood give valuable information to solve the riddle of abdominal diseases. The measurement of the level of bilirubin in the patient of jaundice, cholesterol in obese and thyroid hormone in a constipated patient gives critical information.

The special tests of blood by ELISA techniques (Enzyme Linked Immuno-sorbent Assay) help in diagnosing tuberculosis, hydatid disease and hepatitis 'B' etc.

4. RADIOLOGY & IMAGING TEST

The science of radiology and imaging began with the development of X-ray technique by a German Scientist Willhelm Conrad Roentgen in the year 1895. Subsequently in late twentieth century various new imaging techniques like Ultrasonography, CT scan and M.R.I. became available for general mass. All these techniques provide us with the pictures of body organs which help in differentiating abnormal from normal.

A. Plain X-Ray Abdomen

When a person suffers from abdominal pain, the plain X-Ray image of the abdomen shows the presence of stone in the urinary tract or even gall bladder. It has been found that about 90% stones of urinary tract (kidneys, ureter, bladder etc.) and 10% of gall bladder stones are radio opaque, and are revealed in plain x-ray film of the abdomen.

It is essential that bowel is free from gas and faecal matter while taking X-Ray picture of the abdomen, so that stones and other findings are not obscured. Generally a few medicines are given to the patient prior to taking abdominal X-rays in order to make abdomen free from gas.

B. Barium X-Ray

Gastrointestinal tract is a muscular tube extending from mouth to anus. Its parts are esophagus, stomach, duodenum, ileum, colon and rectum. Imaging study after ingestion of solution of barium is done to evaluate its abnormalities.

'Barium swallow' examination is carried out to investigate food pipe i.e. esophagus. It reveals narrowing, ulcers, dilatation and tumors of the esophagus.

'Barium meal and follow through study' is done to find the diseases of stomach and ileum.

The images of colon are taken by instilling barium sulphate solution through the rectum, known as barium enema examination.

All these studies are carried out in X-Ray suite under expert supervision of a Radiologist. The barium solution is radio-opaque and as it outlines the lumen of gut tube, images are seen on fluoroscopy and recorded on X-ray films. The interpretation of findings of barium studies requires the services of an expert on the subject.

2. ULTRASONOGRAPHY (Synonyms-USG, Ultrasound, Sonography, Echography, Sonar Exam)

Ultrasonography (USG) is a simple, safe, painless and cost-effective imaging technique, which provides quality pictures of the organs inside the abdomen. The probe, a part of the machine, when put on surface of the belly, sends its high frequency sound waves which reflect back from various interfaces. The strength of the returning sound waves are analysed and images are constructed with the help of a complex computerized process. The doctor doing the test observes the images, tries to find out the abnormalities in them and decides about the disease.

In the patients of Jaundice, its cause can be deduced by analyzing the images of liver, gall bladder, bile duct and pancreas etc. It can be judged whether it is caused by edema of the liver (Hepatitis) or due to obstruction in the bile duct through which bile passes from the gall bladder to the duodenum

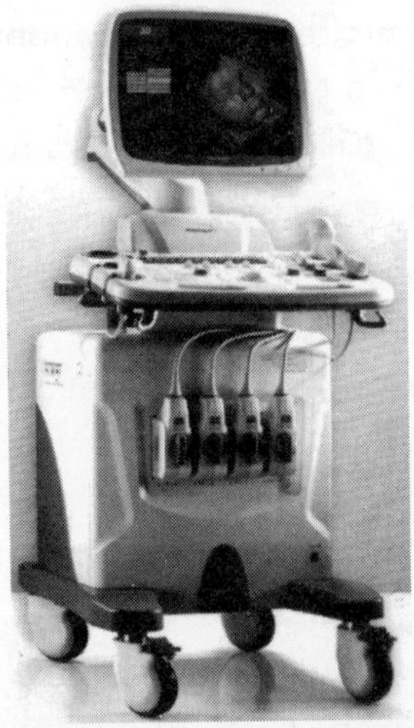

Fig.-12-Ultrasonography Machine

USG provides accurate information about the presence of stones in the gall bladder, kidneys and urinary bladder, abscess and tumors in liver, edema in pancreas and masses in various organs of the abdomen. It can detect even small quantities of abnormal fluid in the abdomen (Ascites) or around the lungs (Pleural Effusion) and heart (Pericardial Effusion).

USG is the preferred imaging modality to assess growth and organ development of the fetus in a pregnant woman. It is used to exclude any birth defects in the child in the womb. It clearly demonstrates majority of the structures of the fetus from its head to toe. As USG can distinctly show all the organs of the fetus, many parents want to know the sex of the fetus from the USG operator. We must realize that detecting and disclosing the sex of the fetus is illegal and it is criminal act under PNDT Act (Pre-natal diagnostic technique act). The Ultrasonologist as well as the attendants of the pregnant women (Husband, In-laws etc) may be punished for this offence.

Fluid collections in abdominal cavity or other spaces can be aspirated under USG guidance and the biochemical analysis of the fluid may provide diagnostic information.

3. C.T. Scan & M.R.I. (Computerized Axial Tomography and Magnetic Resonance Imaging)

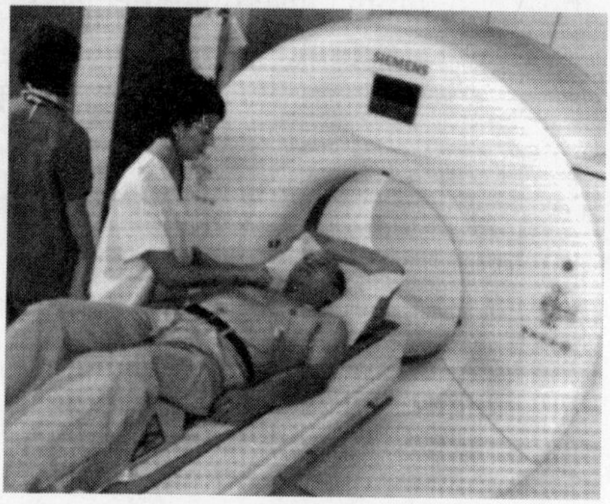

Fig.-13 : CT Scan Machine

These modern imag-ing techniques give ex-cellent cross sectional images of the organs. These provide us re-constructed images of the organ to allow three dimensional assessment of the lesion in the organs.

In cases of cancers of intra-abdominal organs the extent and local spread of the disease, the involvent of lymph nodes and presence of distant spread (metastasis) can be evaluated with CT Scan and MRI tests.

A special protocol with MRI technique known as MRCP (Magnetic Resonance Cholangio Pancreato-graphy) gives excellent images of the bile duct, helping in detecting stone and tumour in it. MRCP test is gradually replacing ERCP test (Endoscopic Retrograde Cholangio Pancreatography) in which, a pipe like endoscope is passed through food pipe upto duodenum. Though ERCP technique is a bit uncomfortable to the patient compared to MRCP, with the former, therapeutic procedures such as extraction of stone from CBD and stenting of blocked CBD can also be performed.

In pregnant women with abdominal pain MRI is recommended in which ultrasound has not identified the cause of patients symptom. CT scan is not done in pregnant women, as the X-Ray radiation may harm the fetus. New innovations in Ultrasonography (Colour Doppler Sonography, Contrast Sonography and Elastography) and in CT Scan (Angiography and Venography) give quite detailed information about health and disease of body organs.

Newer imaging techniques (PET-Position-emission-tomography, SPECT-Single Photon Emission Computed Tomography) give information about both structure and function of various body organs.

4. Endoscopy

Endoscope denotes the genre of equipments which help in visualizing internal organs (Endo-Internal, scope range of view) some examples are:

Organ		**Name of Scope**
Stomach and Duodenum	-	Gasto-duodenoscope
Intestine	-	Ileoscope
Sigmoid colon	-	Sigmoidoscope
Whole colon	-	Colonoscope
Joint	-	Arthroscope
Ear	-	Otoscope
Urinary Bladder	-	Cystoscope

Gasto-duodenoscope is used to observe the lumen of food-pipe, stomach and duodenum. In this instrument a thin flexible fibre-optic telescope is passed through the mouth, down into the intestine. As the tube is flexible its tip can be turned to any direction and throw cool light on corresponding part of gut.

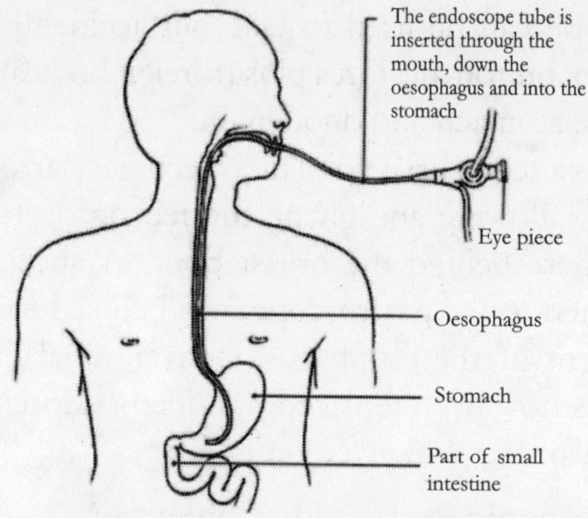

Fig.-14A : Upper gastro-intestinal Endoscope

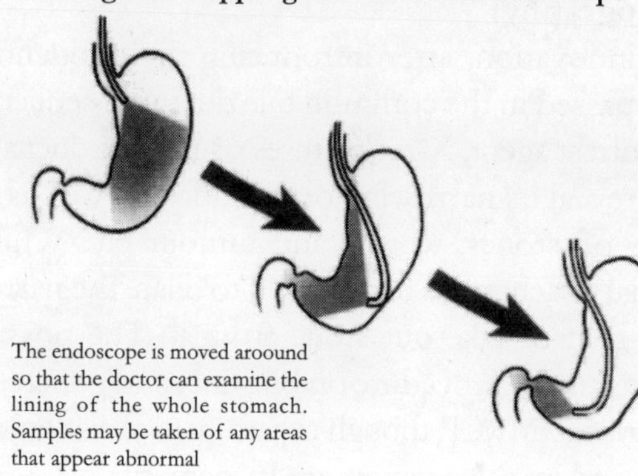

Fig.-14B : Endosopy

We may, with the help of gastro scope see the edema and ulcers in the lining of the esophagus, stomach and duodenum. Tumour like nodules can be detected and tissue for biopsy can be extracted.

Gastroscope can also be utilized for treatment purpose also. In long standing (chronic) disease of the liver, the veins at the junction of esophagus and stomach get dilated (Varices) and blood may ooze from them. Bleeding from these dilated vessels can be stopped and prevented by injecting some medicines in them (Sclerotherapy) or putting rubber bands over swollen vessels (Banding).

Gastroscope can be used to take out accidently ingested things like coin, button, destores pins (foreign bodies) etc, from the esophagus, stomach and duodenum.

Sometimes a segment of food pipe becomes narrow causing difficulty in swallowing and giving the feeling of food being stuck somewhere behind the breast bone. A special type of balloon attached to the gastroscope may be used to dilate the narrow segment of the esophagus. Conventional Fibre-optic endoscope has now been replaced by Video-endoscope which is thinner in diameter and giver better images.

ERCP (Endoscopic Retrograde Cholangio Pancreaticography)

In this innovation, after introducing the duodenoscope a thin tube is passed in the common bile duct .Subsequently after injecting contrast agent, X-ray pictures of the bile duct are taken, which may reveal its narrowing or dilatation as well as absence or presence of stones, worms and tumour etc. While doing ERCP special attachments can be used to dilate the narrow tube, put a stent in it or take out stone from it. The possibility of carrying a treatment procedure on bile duct and pancreas makes ERCP superior to MRCP, though exposure to radiation, injection of contrast and invasive nature are its demerits.

SIGMOIDOSCOPY AND COLONOSCOPY

In this Endoscopic procedure, endoscope (the flexible pipe) is passed through rectum i.e. back passage. Sigmoidoscope is smaller in length and only lower third of colon can be studied where as with Colonoscope the entire length of colon with some part of terminal ileum can also be observed.

Apart from diagnosing diseases of the colon, it can be used to remove polyps from the luminal wall of the colon. Polyps, small lumps which grow and hang from the wall of the colon are quite common in the aged persons of western countries. As some of these polyps may turn into cancerous growth, regular colonoscopic removal of polyps is a routine medical practice in

Europe and America. In our country children suffering bleeding per anus may have rectal polyps which are benign tumours and can be managed by endoscopic polypectomy.

While doing colonoscopy a polyp is trapped in a sling (snare) and then detached from the wall by using electric current, which also seals the bleeding vessel. The polyp thus removed is examined under microscope by a histopathologist to rule out any cancerous changes.

ENDOSONOGRAPHY

Endosonography is a unique innovation in which sonographic imaging system is attached to the tip of the endoscope. As the endoscope is introduced in food pipe and moved onwards, images of tissues around esophagus, stomach and duodenum can be taken.

It has proved quite useful in diagnosing tumors of esophagus, stomach and pancreas and detecting stones in common bile duct. Endosonography is used to aspirate or biopsy from masses in upper gastrointestinal tract,and draining collections around pancreas. Chronic pain of pancreatitis can be managed by use of endosonography instrument.

FEW ILLUSTRATIVE CASES

The advances in science and technology are influencing every aspect of modern life including the practice of medicine. The application of technology in diagnosing and treating abdominal problem has many miraculous outcomes. Some examples are here:-

(A) Mrs. Mala, a young woman had one day severe pain in upper half of belly. She was restless with pain and had vomited many times without any relief. Doctors suspected stones in the gall bladder, which got confirmed on Ultrasonography examination and additionally she was found to have few stones also in the bile duct.

She was sent to the care of gastroentrologist, who did her endoscopic examination. With help of the duodenoscope the mouth of the common bile duct was opened up and stone from it was taken out with special forceps. After two days she underwent surgery for removal of the stone filled gall bladder by key-hole surgery technique (Laparoscopy). She was spared an open operation on abdomen, which gives a large cut and subsequent scar on the abdominal wall and long hospitalisation.

(B) The other person, sixty year old lady had severe jaundice, caused by blockage of the bile duct as a result of infiltration by the cancer at gall bladder neck. The cancer had spread to distant places as she had nodules in liver, enlarged lymph nodes and fluid in abdomen. She had lost her appetite and the itching in skin was intolerable. Surgery was not feasible at this advanced stage of cancer.

The specialist did her endoscopy examination and passed first a guide wire and then a thin tube in the narrow bile duct, thereby restoring the flow of bile. She was relieved of jaundice and itching and quality of her remaining life was improved.

(C) The third example is a six year old child who had inadvertently ingested a coin. Endoscopy revealed the coin, trapped at narrow lower end of food pipe and partially blocking it.

The coin was caught with the help of minute forceps passed through endoscope and was slowly taken out. The method can be used to remove buttons, seeds, fish-bone, tablets and many other accidently ingested things.

Few decades ago the only way to deal with such types of medical problems, was to perform major surgery. Today many major surgeries are avoided by using specialized tools .It is true, modern techniques and equipments have drastically changed and simplified the diagnosis and treatment.

CHAPTER-12

• DIET AND BENEFITS OF VEGETARIANISM

A nutritious and balanced diet is essential to keep us healthy, energetic and free from diseases. Balanced diet consists of food items having carbohydrate, fat, protein, minerals, vitamins and water in proper proportions. It should be adequate in quantity for our current needs as well as to create reserve for the requirements of the future.

Carbohydrate present in cereals provides us energy, where as proteins present in pulse, milk, egg etc help in building new and repair damaged tissue. Fat acts as a reserve store for energy. Vitamins and minerals keep the cells healthy and help us fight diseases.

Our body needs different quantities of various components of a balanced food at various stages of life. The body of an infant and child grows up to an age of 18-20 years, hence it requires more of protein to synthesize new tissues (Anabolism). A healthy active adult, who has to keep his body weight stable, needs mainly carbohydrates for energy. The body generally remains in a state of balance between the ages of 20 to 50 years. Above the age of 50 years when breakdown of tissues (Catabolism) is greater, more protein is required to repair the wear and tear.

A new born child is fully dependent on mother's milk for nutrition. The child needs good amount of protein for the growth of the brain. The diet of the mother requires special attention during pregnancy and lactation as she is practically nourishing two lives. The diet of the mother during this period should have enough pulses, milk, vegetables and fruits. Only a healthy mother can give birth to a healthy child and maintain health during infancy.

The digestive system of our body breaks the complex particles of food into simple molecules, absorbs them and discards the waste part in the stool. The long tube of the alimentary canal has to work hard to perform these functions.

The food digests better when taken relaxingly in a calm and comfortable atmosphere, provides more energy and gives greater psychological satisfaction. Eating in hurry should be avoided. The quantity of food should be in accordance with the requirement of our body. We must realise that the food is needed to sustain life, but the life is not meant for taking food only.

We must know that overeating is an invitation to ill health. Food should be well cooked and simple. Very spicy and fatty foods harm our body. Plain and simple food taken in small quantities is elixir for life.

Obesity which has acquired epidemic like status among affluent people is a result of excessive consumption of fatty food. Quantity of food consumed should be as per our energy requirement .Food should not be taken for entertainment and enjoyment.

It becomes difficult to assimilate fatty and heavy foods (like *Pulao, Paratha, Puree* and non-vegetarian items etc), in diseases of the digestive system. Patients of jaundice, gastroenteritis, enteric fever etc, should be given easily digestible and preferably semisolid foods like *Khichri,* overcooked rice, horlicks and milk. Patients of tuberculosis of gut may take liquid food during initial few days of treatment. Patients of peptic ulcer may benefit from a food having less spices.

We should remember that as walking and running requires muscular activity and spending of energy, so is the case with digesting and assimilating food by the digestive tract. Therefore, larger quantity of food will require greater amount of work by the digestive system.

DIET OF CHILDREN

Young children, who do not have fully developed teeth, simply go on swallowing the food, instead of properly chewing it. Therefore, they should be given well cooked or rather overcooked food, preferably mashed with hand. Children need food more frequently, though in small quantity, therefore, they should not be compelled to eat in rigorous 'three meals a day' manner. They feed better when served in playful manner. It is unwise to impose dining table manners to young children.

While preparing food especially vegetables, the serving meant for children should be put aside before adding spices and chilies etc. If the child is fed with spoon, one should carefully ensure that the food is only warm and not hot.

VEGETARIANISM

When a person relies only on food items sourced from plants, he is labelled as a 'Vegetarian'. The only exceptional item sourced from animals in their diet is milk. Very strict and true 'Vegans' do not even take milk to stay exclusively vegetarian.

The human body including teeth, stomach and entire digestive system is more suited for vegetarian food. The pointed teeth in our mouth, canine are small, which are generally quite large in carnivorous animals like dogs and tigers.

In Britain, few decades back the cows, which are grass eating animals, were fed upon meat to make them grow fast. It led to destruction of their brain cells and they suffered from 'Mad-

Cow Disease'. The human beings who took beef from these animals also suffered brain damage and became victims of 'Creutzfeldt-Jacob Disease'.

Digestion and assimilation of vegetarian food is easier compared to non-vegetarian food. Food that is abundant in green leafy vegetables, fruits and salad are best for human beings. The food of an adult person must consist of at least half a kilogram of fruits, salads and vegetables. Germinated red-gram and soya etc. should be taken raw to get full benefits of vitamins present in them. Cooking germinated red-gram destroys part of its vitamin content.

Fruits & vegetables are low in calorie content and high in fibre; thereby provide a feel of fullness and satiety without adding weight. Their fibre component stimulates intestine and relieves constipation. High fibre food digests slowly and thereby spikes in blood sugar level are avoided. One should develop habit of taking fruits 1-2 hours prior to lunch and dinner, as it well help in keeping the body weight in control by reducing the quantum of food in lunch and dinner.

Coloured pigment of foods (Flavinoids)

The colour of the fruits and vegetables is due to presence of phytochemicals knows as flavinoids. These colour pigments are quite useful for our body as they destroy harmful free radicles formed during biochemical reactions of metabolism.

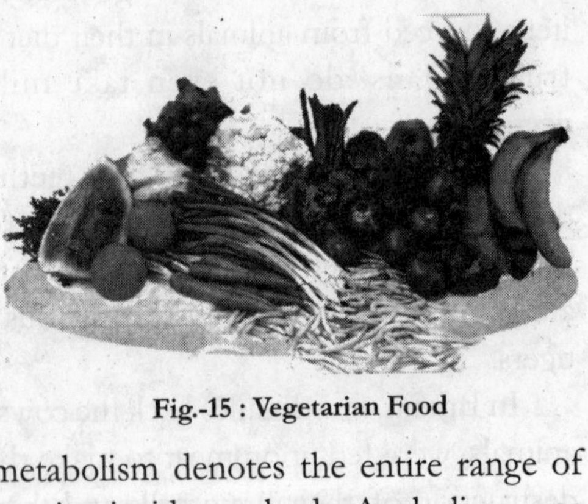

Fig.-15 : Vegetarian Food

The expression, metabolism denotes the entire range of biochemical processes going inside our body. Anabolism, one of its aspects involves digestion, absorption and assimilation of food leading to formation of chemicals needed to build cells and tissue. This is constructive aspect of metabolism. The destructive aspect, knows as catabolism signifies ageing and destruction of cells and damage to the tissues.

Flavinoids induce anabolism and support growth in height and weight of children. Children fed on papaya, tomato, cucumber, mango and green vegetables attain better height and health in long term.

Flavinoids also discourage catabolic processes which weaken our tissue and bodies. In menopausal women, female hormones decrease leading to weakening of body and the bones. In such women the color pigments of food act as hormonal supplement and strengthen her muscles and body.

The flavinoid lycopene present in tomato, beta-carotene in orange and carrot and anthrocyanine in strawberry boost our immunity. Sulpheron, a flavinoid present in cabbage and cauliflower have anticancer property.

Green vegetables like peas, beans, pumpkin etc have plenty of flavinoids in the form of Luteine and Xanthenes. These also contain good quantity of iron and vitamin 'C'.

Consuming plenty of foods and vegetables is essential for the good health of entire family.

Fruits or Fruit Juice?

A question, frequently asked is whether fruits as such are better for health or the juice extracted from them?

When we eat fruit, the cellulose fibre present in it is also ingested which gives bulk to the stool and relieves constipation. It has been found that high fibre diet saves us from cancers of colon.

Eating fruit fills our stomach and gives a feeling of fullness and satiety, thereby reducing the quantity of main meal. This helps in keeping body weight in control.

The fruit juice especially when it is sweetened with sugar contains greater amount of calorie. We can not eat one kilogram apple at one time, however it is quite easy to drink 200ml apple juice extracted out of it, which contains equivalent amount of calorie.

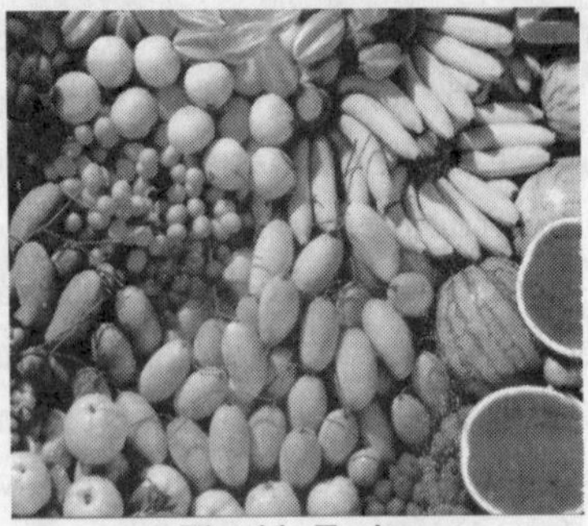

Fig.-16 : Fruits

Eating fruits lets the muscles of face and cheek exercise; it massages and strengthens the gums.

The bottled fruit juices available in markets contain coloring and flavoring agents apart from preservatives. These chemicals are not very safe for our body.

Above mentioned facts imply that consumption of fruits as such is better compared to taking fruit juice. It does not mean that fruit juice is not good for health. Fruit juices also are good for health.

While extracting juice of fruits one should take utmost care to maintain the cleanliness of utensils and equipments like juicer.

Persons suffering from hyperacidity and heartburn should avoid juices of orange, lemon and *mausambi* (sweat lime) which contain large amount of citric acid.

Fruits or Veggies

Fruits and vegetables both contain fibres, phyto-chemicals and flavinoids and are good for health. However, fruits generally are costlier and their availability also is quite limited. Our diet must contain both but with larger quantity of vegetables.

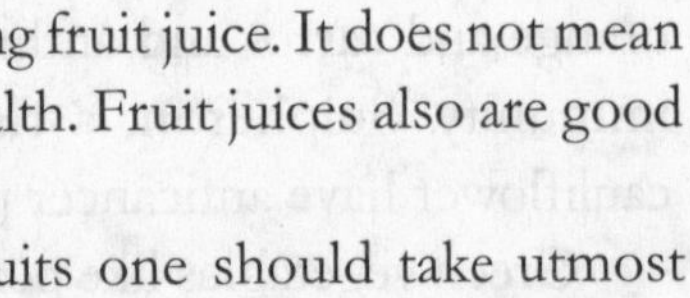

Fig.-17 : Fruits and Vegetables

It is wrong to think that fruits, as they are costlier, are better for health. Also one should not expect greater health benefits from exotic and imported fruits, though their unique taste can be relished. One must take seasonal fruits like mango, guava, papaya and carrots etc when their cost is reasonable.

UTENSILS

The kitchen utensils in past were made from iron, copper and brass like metals. With the changing times the utensils of steel, aluminum and teflon-coatings have come in vogue. Today plastic, ceramic and glass utensils are also being used especially while cooking in microwave ovens.

At least a few household utensils used in cooking food *(Tava, Kadai, Kalchi)* should be made of cast-iron. During the process of cooking, a minute amount of iron goes in food which helps in improving the Haemoglobin level in our blood. This benefit is not accorded by steel utensils.

Aluminium and Teflon vessels should be used only when they are of very high quality. Poor quality utensils of aluminium and Teflon shed minute quantities of metal and chemical respectively, which may be harmful for human body.

Some people use jugs and glasses made of copper to store and drink water. Copper ion is thought to have antibacterial property. Minute amounts of copper and some other elements like zinc and magnesium are considered good for health. These are present in various items of food especially vegetables.

WATER

Water is the medium through which toxic waste products of metabolism are excreted away from the body in the form of urine. It helps keep skin moist and stool soft. A normal healthy adult should take approx 8-10 glasses of water (1.5-2.0 liters) every day, increasing it to 2-3 liters in the summer season.

The deficit of water in the body makes us exhausted and lethargic. The exhaustion and weakness generally experienced in afternoons is due to deficiency of water and electrolytes in the body.

When plain water is not palatable, few drops of lemon or a slice of orange can be put to add flavour. Some fruits like melon, orange, pears contain good quantity of water.

Coconut water has plenty of potassium and other useful minerals in it. Coconut water is a good supplement to replace potassium lost in sweat during summer and in faeces during an attack of diarrhoea.

Coconut tree are abundant in areas like sea-shore where people undergo severe perspiration due to high humidity in the atmosphere. The merciful nature has provided the flora of the kind which human beings need in a particular climatic zone.

Common Salt

Common salt (sodium chloride) is an essential additive to make the food tasty. Sodium is also present in baking soda (Sodium Bicarbonate). It retains fluid in the body and maintains the blood pressure.

Excessive intake of sodium in various forms may cause high blood pressure. Communities consuming lower amounts of salt, have lower average blood pressure.

We should use common salt in moderation, approximately 4-6gms a day. Food products like pickles, *papad,* chips, and packed wheat flour have high quantity of sodium salt. Salads, corn and pea-nuts etc should be sprinkled with lemon juice & black pepper instead of salt, to make tangy. Use of common salt, should generally be restricted to minimal possible amount.

Patient having edema and ascites should drastically reduce salt under the supervision of his doctor.

Persons having low blood pressure, feeling weakness, exhaustion and those who have suffered bouts of loose motion may be advised to take common salt in soup.

CURD (YOGURT)

Consumption of curd helps to keep our intestines healthy. It contains a useful organism Lactobacillus which checks the proliferation of harmful bacteria, E-coli in the intestine. Lactobacillus also helps in synthesing group 'B' vitamins.

Persons who experience breathlessness and asthma on consuming curd should limit or avoid its intake. Curd should be garnished with black pepper or coriander powder rather than common salt in order to avoid blood pressure causing effect of sodium.

TEA

Tea is a healthy beverage when taken in limited quantity (2-3 cups a day). This contains an alkaloid 'Quercetin' which removes harmful chemicals from the body.

Tea stimulates the mind and energizes the body. However, when taken in large quantity it may cause acidity, heart burn, increase in heart rate and disturbs sleep.

A few tea spoonful of milk or a few drops of lemon juice should always be put in the cup of tea as these additives precipitate the undesirable compound Tannin present in tea and make it absolutely safe.

SPICES

The use of a variety of spices is a peculiarity of Indian culinary. The spices improve the digestibility of food, kill germs and also boost our immune system.

Dry spices like ground coriander, turmeric, black pepper, chillies, fenugreek and ginger etc have medicinal properties. Spices should be put in limited quantity, otherwise it will mask the original taste of the foods and vegetables.

TURMERIC

The yellow color of turmeric is due to presence of the pigment cucuramin which has antibacterial properties. The beneficial effects of poultices of turmeric and lime on blunt injuries and foot sprain is well recognised.

Turmeric is absolutely safe for the patient of jaundice. It is a myth that turmeric causes and deepens the jaundice which in majority of the patients is due to viral infection.

CHILLIES

The alkaloid capsaicin present in green and red chilies, increase the flow of blood to the intestines, thereby aid digestion. It contains good quantity of vitamin C.

Excessive consumption of chilies may cause burning in abdomen, heartburn, acidity and may aggravate peptic ulcer.

GINGER

Ginger is considered home remedy for cold and cough. Drinking Ginger tea in winters prevents from bad effects of cold on lungs. Gingerone, the chemical present in Ginger has antibacterial properties.

ONION

Onion and garlic reduce the deposition of cholesterol on the internal lining of blood vessels, prevent the clogging of lumen and protect us from heart and brain attacks. Many *Vaishnav hindus* and *Jains* do not consume onion etc due to religious beliefs.

Quantity of Food Intake

The calorie requirement of a person depends upon his physical activities as mental work does not spend much energy. Mental work may exhaust someone but it does not increase the calorie demands of the body. Labourers and field workers require greater amount of calorie compared to an office worker.

We must realise that the muscles and glands of the gastrointestinal tract have to work to masticate, digest, propel and absorb the food. It implies that simple food will easily be digested compared to a heavy and fatty meal. When large quantity of high fatty food stays in gut, it causes bloating, gas and constipation. In other words, overeating is an important cause of abdominal discomforts.

Light meal gives rest to the gut and body. Occasional skipping of meal, replacing cereals with fruits and reducing salt content, help in avoiding abdominal problems. As the children are growing, they may need greater amount of calorie compared to a grown up adults.

To think that greater quantity of food will give us more energy is fallacious. Exhaustion and tension can not be alleviated with food. Majority of the people consider food a way of entertainment and enjoy a range of delicacies in parties and ceremonies. The quantity of food taken should be guided by our physical activity and not by its availability. During celebrations, when variety of food is offered, only small amounts should be taken to relish the taste. Overeating is an invitation to abdominal problems.

Our motto should be **"Eat for living"** and not **"live for eating"**.

Interval of Food Intake

Generally we take three major meals a day; breakfast, lunch and dinner. Children with their growing bodies, and elderly people with weak digestive systems, may take their overall amount of food divided into five or six portions a day. A sick person should be allowed small amounts of easily digestible food at 2-3 hours interval.

Adults having normal body weight should marginally under eat to keep the weight in control. The diet of adults should be limited and should not be tummy full.

A working adult should take good breakfast, containing about 40% of his calorie requirement of the day. The lunch should be medium with 30% of the calorie. Dinner should be light with 20% of energy needs and rest 10% calorie is supplied by snacks etc. The dinner should be taken at least two hours before going to bed, in order to avoid gastro-esophageal reflux and its consequences.

The home made Indian lunch is an excellent example of wholesome and complete food. The roti and boiled rice in Indian thali supply carbohydrates, *daal* (lentil soup) and *dahi* (yogurt) give protein and a teaspoonful of *ghee* give fat. Vitamins and minerals are provided by vegetables and salads. *Chutney, papad,* pickles and spices aid digestion and make the food tasty. It is not an exaggeration to say that "Indian *thali* is best food in the world".

ORGANIC FOOD

Modern agriculture practices involve extensive uses of chemical fertilizers to improve the yield. Chemical pesticides and insecticides are sprayed to protect the crops from pests and insects respectively. These inorganic chemicals enhance the production and help meet the demand of food of the growing world population. However these chemicals ingested through food are harmful for our body system. Some scientific studies suggest excess quantity of insecticides in soil and food is responsible for increased incidence of cancers in the Gall Bladder in transgangetic belt.

The produce of crops raised without using chemicals and fertilisers is labelled as 'organic food'. Such food is considered healthier and safer for body system. However, powder made from dried *neem* leaves can be used to save crop from insects and cow-dung can be mixed in soil to enhance yield of the organic food.

Organic food is generally costlier, which acts a dampener for its wide spread uses. The awareness regarding organic food is increasing and it will surely lead to availability of better quality food.

FASTING

People fast for two reasons:

1. Religious purpose - as a gesture to worship God.
2. Weight Reduction.

1. Fasting as a ritual of religious worship

Hindus fast on the occasions of *Chhath, Janamasthmi, shivratri* and *Ekadashi* etc. Hindu women fast on the occasion of *Karwa Chouth,* praying for longer lives of their husband.

Majority of the Muslims go for day fasting during their holy month of Ramjan. During this month they breakfast after sunset and take limited quantity of food before sunshine.

Whatever be the religious implication of fasting, it disturbs the fine tuning of the digestive system. Hunger may initiate hunger pain and abdominal cramps. The release of bile, without the presence of food may irritate gut causing pain and vomiting. Reduced intake of water may cause dehydration, leading to lethargy, weakness and exhaustion. The control of blood sugar levels and co-ordination with medications gets disturbed in diabetics. All these factors prompt us to discourage fasting. When fasting is a compulsion, at the least water and fruits *(Falahar)* should be allowed.

2. For weight reduction

Fasting is never justified for weight reduction. Occasional skipping of food generally is followed by overeating which compensates for reduction in calorie during fasting.

In order to become slim a person has to reduce calorie intake in all meals and increase calorie burning by physical activity, consistently for a long period. Weight reduction is a long drawn process. Occasional fasting is meaningless for this objective.

Fat is an essential component of our food. In an average diet, about 20 percent calorie is provided by fat in food. It also supplies some vitamins like 'A', 'D' and 'K' which are fat soluble vitamins. An absolute refusal of fat intake for the purpose of weight reduction may harm the body.

CHAPTER-13

• PRECAUTION WITH MEDICATION

Medicines have become integral part of modern life. Large numbers of persons are on long term medications to control blood pressure and blood sugar levels, to prevent heart attack, to reduce cholesterol level and to supplement vitamins and hormones. Medicines for minor problems like simple headache are easily available over the counter of the shops without a medical prescription. Our society has acquired a 'pill popping culture'.

Excessive consumption of pain killers like aspirin, nimuselide and diclofenac and steroids can injure the internal lining of the stomach and duodenum leading to ulcer formation. The probability of harm is greater if pain-killers are taken on empty stomach. Therefore pain-killer medicine should always be taken after ingesting some food.

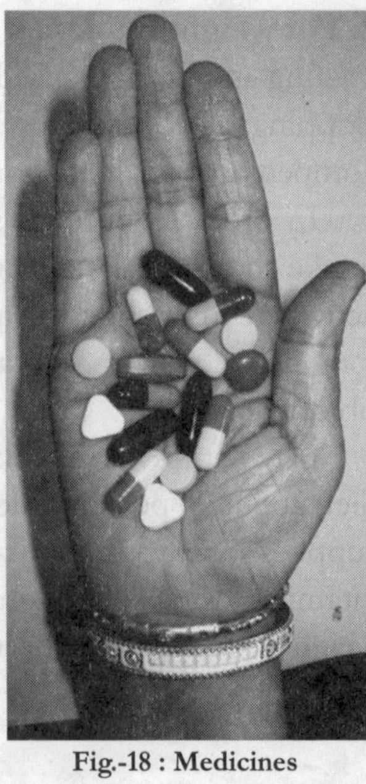

Fig.-18 : Medicines

The capsule and tablets may be arrested at the narrow region at the junction of food pipe and stomach (Gastro-esophageal Junction). These should always be swallowed with about half a glass of water, so that they can pass easily into the stomach. A gulp of water should be taken to moisten the inner lining of esophagus followed by the tablet and few sips of water. The water dissolves the contents of the tablets and capsules, thereby sparing stomach from damage due to direct contact. Dissolution in water also improves absorption and facilitates excretion of metabolites in the urine.

A doctor is supposed to guide the patient about the quantity, timing and duration of taking medicines. He is expected to instruct clearly whether a given medicine is to be taken on empty stomach or after food.

When someone is taking medicines prescribed by more than one doctor, he should show all the prescription to them so that repetition and harmful drug interactions may be avoided. This dictum applies also when medicines of more than one system (Allopathy, Homeopathy, Ayurvedic and Unani etc) are being taken.

PREVENTION OF MEDICAL PROBLEMS

Physical activities like walking, jogging, swimming and aerobic exercises are very essential to keep us fit and healthy. Physical exercise improves the circulation of entire body including muscles and brain. They strengthen the muscles, boost immunity and make the body strong. Exercises trim the flabbiness and make skin taut and face glow. An adult should spend at least one hour on alternate days in gymnasium or playground. One should begin the day with morning walk at the time of sunrise. These simple health promoting facts are well recognised and known to everyone. But how many people practice it?

The inventions of modern science and innovations of modern life, are curtailing the demand of physical activity. Many household appliances; washing machine, dish washers and vacuum cleaners are doing physical work on behalf of human beings. Bikes, cars, lifts and escalators are making legs a spare item. People are becoming overweight and obese.

Yog asnas and Relaxation techniques and *Pranyam* improve physical as well as mental health.

In order to improve the health status of population, a collective effort is needed. Twenty to thirty minutes time may be allocated in schools, colleges and offices for physical actively.

Morning walk in residential areas and physical training in student hostels should be promoted.

CHAPTER-14

• MISCELLANEOUS CONDITIONS

(A) ASCITES

The box like cavity of abdomen in which various organs liver, spleen and intestines are located is known as peritoneal cavity. A thin layer of fluid is present normally in this cavity. Ascites is an abnormal accumulation of fluid in the abdominal cavity.

Diseases of many organs like that of heart, kidneys, liver and also malnutrition may cause generalized edema, with swollen feet, puffy eyelids and ascites. In our country hepatitis, cirrhosis of liver, abdominal tuberculosis and kidney failure are important causes of ascites.

Ascites may not be associated with generalised edema like in cases of abdominal tuberculosis. Ascites may be a cause of increase in abdominal girth. Doctors have developed techniques to assess increased amount of fluid in abdomen in clinical examination. Ultrasonography has proved an important tool in detecting ascites, particularity in small amounts.

Ascitic fluid is sometimes aspirated and biochemical examination of the sample is done to reach a diagnosis. Aspiration of ascitic fluid under direct Ultrasonographic observation is safe and avoids inadvertent damage to internal abdominal organs.

(B) DISEASE OF ANUS

The symptoms of most of the diseases affecting anus (back passage) and tissues near it are similar. These symptoms are pain around anus, constipation and appearance of blood in the stool.

1. Anal Fissures-Anal fissures refer to the breaches and ulcers at anus. When hard stool passes out, sometimes it tears the posterior part of anal opening resulting in fissures, which get infected by bacteria. Fissures are quite painful and may lead to bleeding after bowel movement.

2. Piles (Hemorrhoids)-In this condition the veins around anus get congested and swollen and bulge out as berry like masses. These bulging masses cause pain, constipation and inability to pass faeces and gas, which lead to abdominal distension.

Sometimes the swollen veins get ruptured and bleed profusely.

3. Proctitis and Ano-rectal Abscess-Infection of anal canal is termed proctitis .It may lead to the formation of pus pockets in the deeper layers, called ano-rectal abscess. In this condition patient suffers excruciating pain around anus along with constipation and fever.

Apart from these relatively less harmful problems some other serious diseases (tuberculosis and cancer) may affect perianal area.

The correct diagnosis and treatment of diseases around can be achieved only with the services of a specialist –Surgeon or Gastroenterologist. The affected area may need visual and proctoscopic inspection. One should not ignore and conceal such problems out of embarrassment. Visiting quacks for surgical operation is not justified and may lead to complications.

(C) FATTY LIVER

The overall fat content in the bodies of obese people is high. It is deposited at various places such as beneath the skin, at the interfaces of organs inside the abdomen and also within the cells of the liver. On account of increased amount of fat in its cells the size of the liver increases. The fat in the liver also interferes with its function. Excessive fat deposition in liver is considered abnormal and is termed as fatty liver.

Liver is found to be fatty in most of obese people and about half of the patient of diabetes. Alcohol intake for long duration may also lead to fatty liver. Certain other conditions like pregnancy, childhood malnourishment and intestinal bypass operation may also cause fatty liver. Abnormally high ingestion of fruit juices which contain fructose may also cause fatty liver. Fatty liver is a common entity in western countries and certain states of India (Punjab, Gujarat, and Rajasthan) where obesity has acquired endemic status. Fatty liver leads to enlargement of liver and derangement of liver function. It may occasionally progress to cirrhosis of liver and its consequences.

Fatty liver acquires importance because of its association with certain disease, forming a complex, known as Metabolic Syndrome. The components of the metabolic Syndrome are obesity, hypertension, diabetes mellitus and lipid disorders. A large number of such persons have fatty liver also.

The awareness about fatty liver has increased due to availability of high quality ultrasound equipments. It provides excellent clinical grade images of liver for correct interpretation of various diseases. Recently some medicines which claim reduction in the fat content of liver also have been approved for dispensing.

The most effective measure to avoid fatty liver is to keep the body weight within normal range. Increased physical activity, exercises, *yoga,* regular intake of fruits, vegetables and salads, and avoidance of fatty food and overeating may save us from developing fatty liver.

(D) IRRITABLE BOWEL SYNDROME (IBS)

Some people, who otherwise appear to be quite healthy, incessantly complain of abdominal pain, diarrhoea, constipation and abdominal distension. In spite of having abdominal problems for months to years, they do not lose weight and have quite good energy level. Extensive medical work-up of such patients including tests of urine, stool, X-Rays, Ultrasonography, Sigmoidoscopy and Colonoscopy turn out to be absolutely normal. Doctors denote this condition by the term 'Irritable Bowel Syndrome'.

We know that some people are temperamentally irritable and complaining type. They overreact to the ordinary events of life. An analogy may thus be made that some bowels over react to certain foods or drinks or stressful events of life. Generally such persons also suffer from nervousness, depression, inferiority complex, anxiety, fear for the unknown and other psychological symptoms. Some of them nurture fear of developing cancer (Cancer phobia). The patients of IBS though not suffering from any harmful disease process appears to be lost and helpless.

Patient of IBS do not suffer fever, loss of appetite, loss of weight and appearance of blood in the stool. Presence of these symptoms generally indicates presence of some other disease.

Management of IBS is complex and has to be done at two levels.

At one level the patient is given medicines to provide relief in symptoms of constipation, diarrhoea and abdominal pain. The patient is encouraged to identify the items in food and beverages which trigger and aggravate the symptoms and avoid them. Increasing whole grains, full bran wheat and fruits; reducing coffee, tea and cola drinks and stopping smoking and alcohol are generally quite helpful. Gas producing foods like reddish, beans, *sattu,* and cucumber etc may be avoided.

The second level of management is to relieve the person of the stress. He has to develop a relaxed temperament and take unpleasant events in day-to-day life sportingly. The pain and constipation in such patients is generally tolerable. However, the reaction to those symptoms is problematic. It creates a vicious cycle of 'pain-stress-more pain' which needs to be disrupted. Yoga, deep breathing exercises, meditation and relaxation techniques may bring remarkable improvement in such persons.

(E) FOOD ALLERGY

Allergy is the reaction of the body to the substances which it dislikes and considers foreign. Allergy to a substance is expressed as rashes, eruptions and wheal. Wheal is a small localised area of redness and swelling, which is seen commonly after ant or bee sting.

Sometimes our body is allergic to food-stuffs, particularly eggs, fishes, shrimps and mushrooms. The body does not like the type of protein present in them. Occasionally the reaction to egg protein may be quite severe leading to breathlessness and choking.

Children may be allergic to bottled and packed food stuffs such as sauces, ketchups, jams and jellies. The chemical substance used as colour, flavour and preservative in packed food may act as an allergen. Children may complain of abdominal pain on taking allergenic food.

In our part of country allergy to rice, pulses and vegetables are not reported, except occasional instances of allergy to chemicals used in polishing and coloring pulses.

Allergy to food has some geographical variations also. In a population, a small percentage of people may be allergic to the food item most commonly consumed in that area. In Japan where rice is the most common staple food, some people are allergic to it. In Finland, people suffer from allergy to fishes where as in North India few persons are allergic to wheat flour which are, respectively the most commonly taken food items in these parts of the world. The allergy to wheat flour is called coeliac disease.

COELIAC DISEASE

In Northern India some children and adults are allergic to gluten present in the wheat flour. This is a unique example of allergy to a substance present in food made with wheat, barley and oat.

When the infants in age group 6 months to 1 year are switched from mothers' milk to cereals, they begin having diarrhoea and distension of the abdomen. Such children become weak, irritable and suffer poor growth.

Coeliac disease is a genetic disorder and is the result of an abnormal gene in the body. Certain types of blood tests and microscopic examination of tissue taken from duodenum clinches the diagnosis of coeliac disease.

Specific treatment of coeliac disease is not available at present. The affected person has to change his food items and switchover to foods based on rice (boiled rice, idli, *Kheer* etc), pulses *(besan* and *sattu)* and maize. Fruits, vegetables and milk can be taken in plenty, avoiding bread, biscuits, cookies, burger and pizzas etc. Children may sometimes dislike these restrictions, when the food pattern of entire family may need a change so that child accepts it.

We must realise that food allergy is different to food poisoning and Intolerance. Allergy is related to reaction to a specific food product in a few persons. Food poisoning is caused by consuming stale and infected food and affects majority of the persons consuming the unhygienic food. Lactose intolerance is not allergy. It is caused by deficiency of an enzyme (lactase) rather than reaction to milk.

(F) HERNIA

When a tissue or an organ protrudes out of its cavity through a normal or abnormal opening, it is called hernia. Abdomen is a part of body where hernias commonly occur; as it is a large cavity, it keeps many fixed and mobile organs and it has many normal and potential openings. The commonest of all forms of hernias is Inguinal Hernia where a portion of small intestine passes through a tunnel in groin and descends down into the scrotum.

Our abdomen is comparable to a big sac. If some part or lining of the sac becomes weak, the things kept in it will bulge and fall out of it. Similarly if the wall of the abdomen becomes weak at any point the organ will protrude or herniate out through it.

Generally, loops of small intestine pass through abdominal hernia; however stomach, omentum, liver, urinary bladder and ovaries etc. may also herniate.

Hernia is visible as a nodule or bulge which increases on coughing and straining and becomes less prominent or disappears on lying down. Generally the size of the hernia and its opening goes on increasing over a period of years. People attempt to avoid surgery by using medicines, applying pressure from hernia belt and try alternative medicines, without availing any benefit. One has to accept the fact that the hernia can only be repaired by surgery.

The hernias have been classified on various bases. Depending upon the time of onset hernia may be congenital (since birth) or acquired (in later part of life). Depending upon the location it may be Inguinal, Umbilical, epigastric,femoral or hiatus etc. Hernias in front part of the abdomen are ventral hernia and on back side dorsal hernia.

Hernia occurring in the scar of a surgery is termed Incisional Hernia.

CAUSES OF HERNIA

There are two main factors responsible for abdominal hernia - Weakness of the abdominal wall and widening of an opening.

Hernia is promoted by medical problems which increase the pressure inside abdomen such as:

1. Constipation - Person strains at passing stool.
2. Enlarged Prostate - Straining at passing Urine.
3. Cough and breathlessness etc.

Obese people are more prone to hernia as their abdominal wall is fatty but the layer of muscles is thin.

A common hernia in women is the incisional hernia that occurs in the scar of caesarian surgery performed to deliver the child.

PROBLEMS WITH HERNIA

In the initial stages the protruding part of hernia, returns back to its original place when intra abdominal pressure is reduced and is called reducible hernia.

Subsequently the hernia gets stuck in its sac and becomes irreducible. At this stage its blood supply is disturbed and tissue is damaged (strangulation causing gangrene) which is an alarming and emergency situation.

Hernia should ideally be operated when it is reducible.

SURGERY FOR HERNIA

The type of surgery and anesthesia is chosen on the basis of age and health status of the person and the location, size and reducibility of hernia. The advent of Laparoscopic surgery has proved a boon as today the hernia can be repaired by making only a few small holes on the body wall. The size of incision, amount of bleeding and the chances of infection all are drastically reduced by the laparoscopic technique. Sometimes a mesh made of metal or synthetic fibres is put over the defect of hernia to cover it and strengthen the repair.

One should avoid strenuous work after the surgery of abdominal hernia. Ample time should be given for the wound to heal and get strengthened before resuming normal physical activity. During the post operative period of recovery only easily digestible food should be taken. Constipation, urinary obstruction and bronchial asthma, the aggravating factors should be properly managed prior to the surgery of the abdominal hernia.

The problem of hernia should not be taken lightly .The surgery should not be delayed. It becomes quite difficult to repair large hernias and cover the large defects. Delayed surgery becomes an act of testing the skill of the surgeon, which should be avoided.

(G) ABDOMINAL SYMPTOMS IN OTHER MEDICAL CONDITIONS

Some diseases pertaining to other body systems may affect digestive system and cause abdominal discomfort:

1. Diabetes

Diabetes is caused by the deficiency of the hormone insulin produced by the pancreas. The long standing diabetes causes damage to nerves of the body (Diabetic neuropathy).

The activities of the muscles of digestive tract are controlled by nerves. These nerves weaken in long standing diabetes and lead to reduced motility of the gut causing abdominal fullness after meals (Diabetic gastropathy) and constipation (Diabetic Colopathy). There may also be difficulty in swallowing and bloating of abdomen. Some patients of diabetes develop hyperactive intestines leading to diarrhoea and occasional soiling of clothes (involuntary defecation).

2. Thyroid Gland

Thyroxine, the hormone produced by the thyroid gland located in front part of the neck, aids in metabolism and provides energy to the body.

Deficiency of thyroid hormones cause lethargy, weight gain and diminished gut motility leading to constipation.

In contrast, an excess of the thyroid hormone in body makes the person agitated and lose weight. It may increase the motility of gut leading to diarrhoea.

3. Renal Diseases

The main function of the kidneys is to excrete harmful products of the metabolism, urea and creatinine in the urine. In renal diseases, the excretion of these products is hampered leading to rise in their blood levels-uremia. High blood levels of urea and creatinine influence centers in the brain, causing nausea, vomiting and loss of appetite. Uremia may also cause weakness, lethargy, excessive yawning and in advance stages unconsciousness.

Patients of high blood pressure are given low-dose aspirin to decrease the probability of heart attack. A person taking low-dose aspirin has more probability of bleeding from the inner lining of the stomach, if he has associated renal problems. Patients of renal disease should take aspirin and other pain relieving medicines only on the advice of specialist physician.

4. Diseases of Nervous System

Brain and spinal cord, the parts of the nervous system influence the activities of urinary bladder and intestines. The control of these organs is partly voluntary guided by the brain and partly involuntary as a reflex through spinal cord.

Diseases of the nervous system may cause constipation, diarrhoea and involuntary defecation. Paralysis of both legs (Paraplegia) or the paralysis of half of the body (Hemiplegia) may lead to loss of control on passing urine and faeces.

A rise in tension within the skull cavity, termed raised intracranial tension, may cause headache and vomiting.

5. Herpes Zoster

This viral infection manifests as rashes and papules in skin distributed in curvilinear pattern. The virus spreads along the course of nerves beneath the skin. Herpes infection of the abdominal skin may initially cause pain abdomen, before the appearance of rashes. The rashes cause unbearable burning pain in the affected area. Pain may persist for many months after healing of the rashes (post herpetic neuralgia).

(H) FEVER (Pyrexia)

Fever denotes the physical state of body when its temperature goes above the upper limit of normal range of variation. At a higher than normal level of temperature, person feels uneasy, lethargic, thirsty and may have body-ache and headache. The normal range of body temperature in adults is 97-99 degree Fahrenheit (37 degree centigrade). Possibility of fever is considered when temperature begins rising above 99 degree F and becomes definite above 100°F.

Fever is a symptom and not a disease in itself. The temperature of the body may occasionally rise even without a disease. A person may become feverish after unaccustomed physical exercise or during a hot summer afternoon when the outside temperature reaches 110 degree F (44 degree C). One should chart the measurement of mouth temperature taken at six hourly intervals and show it to the doctor to help him decide whether one has fever and what could be its cause.

The rise in body temperature is generally due to release of pyrogens in the blood, which are chemicals released by the destruction of white blood cells while fighting with bacteria and other pathogens. Abdominal diseases like tuberculosis, hepatitis and entero-colitis may cause fever.

Medical services should be urgently sought in following situations:-

1. When the body temperature is rising above 105 degree F.
2. The age of the patient is less than 12 months or above 60 years.
3. Fever has lasted for more than 48 hours.
4. There is stiffness of neck and body or intolerable headache along with fever.

Fever leads to loss of taste and appetite, leading to curtailment of food intake. The high temperature accelerates catabolism causing loss of protein. Long standing fever leads to loss of weight.

Care of a febrile person

The body of the febrile person should repeatedly be wiped with a wet towel to bring down the temperature. Cool water from the tap suffices the purpose. Patient should wear loose clothing to allow air circulation needed for cooling effect. Tight clothing, sweaters and blankets trap the heat generated by body resulting in further rise of temperature.

In malaria, the temperature of the body rises rapidly with shivering. Patient may need to be covered with blankets during this initial phase of rising temperature.

Diet during Fever

A patient having fever may be given liquids and semi solid foods (milk, soup, horlicks, *khichri and kheer* etc). His calorie requirements should be taken care of with easily digestible preparations like *roti, daal,* mashed potato and *rasgullah.* The old proverb, 'starve the fever', is not tenable in modern medical practice. A feverish patient requires more calories due to high metabolic rate.

(I) THE MIND AND THE ABDOMEN

The brain controls the activities of all other organs of body. The size of a human brain is larger as compared to the brains of other animals. The human brain has the capability to think, remember and analyze facts and experience a wide range of emotions such as love, hate, anger, sorrow and jealousy which other animals do not posses. The emotions and thoughts coming up in the brain directly or indirectly influence the working of the heart, lungs as well as abdominal organ.

Everyone has experienced the fast thumping of heart in fear,anger and excitement. Some people rush to toilet on getting bad news as bowels become hyperactive. In sorrow and depression the desire for food is lost, as intestines slow down. Anxiety, irritation and anger increase the secretion of acid in the stomach leading to hyperacidity, heart burn and upper abdominal discomfort. Excess of acid may damage inner lining of stomach causing peptic ulcer. An old medical proverb says that 'Hurry', Worry' and 'Curry' cause peptic ulcers.

Obesity, diabetes and hypertension, the scourges of modern life have causative link with psyche and mind of persons. People have been found to eat more during depression. Eating in such people becomes a means to derive happiness instead of only satiating hunger. Overeating leads to obesity and its consequences.

A positive attitude towards life and people, keeps us mentally and physically fit. A friendly and pleasant demeanour keeps us away from diseases. No one is born happy, but everyone is born with ability to be happy and make others happy by flashing smiles.

We may make ourselves worthier by spending some time, money and energy for the benefit of the poor and downtrodden. We may get rid of anxiety and tension by having faith in God and in our good deeds. Love people around you. Find the good in people and ignore the bad in them. Spread the energy of enthusiasm and light of hopefulness.

Theses measures may not protect you from abdominal diseases like gall stone and T.B., but without doubt they will save you from many discomforts like gas, bloating, heart burn and may be stomachache and constipation. Therefore,

BE HAPPY AND LET OTHERS BE HAPPY.

WEIGHT CHART

Recommend weight for adults above 20 years according to the heights:

Height in cms.	Feet & Inches	Weight Male (kg.)	Weight Female (kg.)
152	5'0"	50.8-54.4	50.8-54.4
155	5'1"	51.7-57.3	51.7-55.3
157	5'2"	56.3-60.3	53.1-56.7
160	5'3"	57.6-61.7	54.4-58.1
162	5'4"	58.9-63.5	56.3-59.9
165	5'5"	60.8-65.3	57.6-61.2
168	5'6"	62.2-66.7	58.9-63.5
170	5'7"	64.0-68.5	60.8-65.3
173	5'8"	65.8-70.8	62.2-66.7
175	5'9"	67.6-72.6	64.0-68.5
178	5'10"	69.4-74.4	65.8-70.3
180	5'11"	71.2-76.2	67.1-71.7
183	6'0"	73.0-78.5	68.5-73.9

INDEX

How to have healthy tummy, healthy body and healthy mind

What to eat?

- Fruits, Vegetables, Salads and whole grains (Puffed rice, *Chura*, Red gram, *Moong, dalia*).

Eat Less:-

- Fatty food (Butter, *Ghee*, Sweets etc.).
- Non-vegetarian food (Eggs, Meat, Fish etc.).

Banned Items:-

- Tobacco (*Pan, Gutkha, Kaini, Bidi,* Cigarrette).
- Alcohol (Beer, Brandy, Whisky etc.).

What to do?

- Exercise, Walking, Swimming, *Yoga, Pranayam.*

What not to do?

- Worry, Hurry, Anger, Anxiety, Greed.

How to live?

- Always smiling, happily living in present.

❑❑❑